HOW TO EAT WHILE LABOUTING AND LIVING

A Guide to Quitting Ultra-Processed Foods for Good

GIANNA POWEL

A *PQ Unleashed* book

DOWNLOAD YOUR FREE E-BOOK

As our way of thanking you for purchasing *How to Eat while Enjoying and Living*, you'll get *Three Highly Effective Communications Strategies* for free! This e-book features three everyday communication strategies to effectively connect with anyone and get them to listen

To get your free e-book, please go to https://pqunleashed.com/howtoeatwhileenjoyingandliving to receive the download instructions.

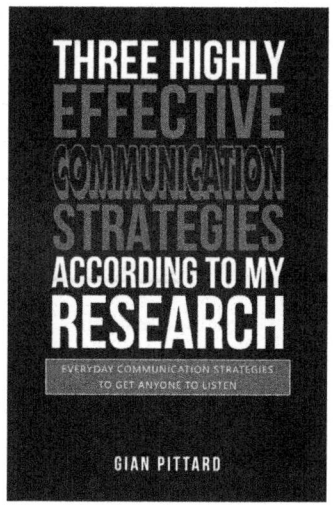

© Copyright 2022 by Mind-Kern Inc. All rights reserved.

Without the prior written permission of the publisher, no part of this publication may be stored in a retrieval system, replicated, or transferred in any form or medium, digital, scanning, recording, printing, mechanical, or otherwise, except as permitted under the 1976 United States Copyright Act, sections 107 and 108. Permission concerns should be directed to the publisher's permission department.

Legal Notice

This book is copyright protected. It is only to be used for personal purposes. Without the author's or publisher's permission, you cannot paraphrase, quote, copy, distribute, sell, or change any part of the information in this book.

Disclaimer

This book is written and published independently. Please keep in mind that the material in this publication is solely for educational and entertainment purposes. All efforts have been made to provide authentic, up-to-date, trustworthy, and comprehensive information. There are no express or implied assurances. The purpose of this book's material is to assist readers in having a better understanding of the subject matter. The activities, information, and exercises are provided solely for self-help information. This book is not intended to replace expert psychological, legal, financial, or other guidance. If you require counseling, please get in touch with a qualified professional.

By reading this text, the reader accepts that the author will not be held liable for any damages, indirectly or directly experienced, due to the information included herein, particularly, but not limited to, omissions, errors, or inaccuracies. As a reader, you are accountable for your decisions, actions, and consequences.

CONTENTS

PQ UNLEASHED INTRODUCTION IX

INTRODUCTION XI
A Brief Chapter by Chapter Breakdown of the Book xiii
    A Book That Is Only Helpful When You Take Action xiv

CHAPTER 1: WHY WE CANNOT GET ENOUGH OF UNHEALTHY FOOD 1
The Food Industry Is Out to Take Your Money 2
    The Big Six 4
    The Bliss Point 11
Your Food Addiction and Dopamine 12
Key Takeaways 14

CHAPTER 2: THE IMPORTANCE OF EATING HEALTHY AND ENJOYING YOUR FOOD 17
Why You Should Eat Healthily 19
Tips to Make Your Food Taste Better 22
A 10-Day Detox Diet Plan 24
    What Are You Going to Eat? 25
    Working Around the Obstacles 29

Key Takeaways 29

CHAPTER 3: THE CONSEQUENCES OF NOT LEADING A HEALTHY LIFESTYLE 31

List of Micronutrients That People Are Commonly Malnourished In 33
- Calcium 34
- Folate 35
- Iodine 35
- Iron 36
- Magnesium 37
- Potassium 38
- Zinc 38
- Vitamin A 39
- Vitamin B6 40
- Vitamin B12 40
- Vitamin C 41
- Vitamin D 42

List of Diseases Caused by Consuming Unhealthy Foods 43
- Obesity 43
- Type 2 Diabetes 45
- Cirrhosis 48
- Chronic Kidney Disease 49
- Heart Disease 50
- Alzheimer's Disease 54
- Cancer 55

Am I Scaring You? 56
Key Takeaways 58

CHAPTER 4: RESEARCH STUDIES ON ENJOYING HEALTHY FOOD 61

Bias Reversal 62
- Bias Reversal in Action 63

Mental Labeling 64

Mental Labeling in Action 66
Memory Rehearsal 68
    Memory Rehearsal in Action 69
Key Takeaways 70

CHAPTER 5: THE CHALLENGES OF EATING HEALTHY AND ENJOYING HEALTHY FOOD....73

Healthy Foods Are More Expensive and Inconvenient to Prepare .74
    Making Healthy Eating Affordable and Easier 75
    It Is Not About Changing Your Conditions 77
Healthy Living Is Difficult if Those Around You Are Not Interested 78
    Bring Your Family and Friends on Board 79
    How Far Would You Go to Protect the Ones You Love To What Lengths Are You Willing to go to Protect Your Family 81
Healthy Living in the Face of Self-Limiting Beliefs 82
    What You Tell Yourself 83
    What You Do Not Say 85
Key Takeaways 87

CHAPTER 6: PRACTICAL TIPS TO EATING HEALTHIER 89

Keep a Food Diary 90
    10-Day Food Journal 91
Practice Mindful Eating 92
    The Raisin Test 94
Be Thoughtful in Choosing Your Diet 95
Do Intermittent Fasting 96
Get Rid of Sugar 98
    Imagine What You Are Consuming 100
Have a Cup of Coffee 101
Do Not Forget to Exercise 104
More Key Tips That We Take for Granted 106
Key Takeaways 108

CONCLUSION 109
What Has Been Keeping You Stuck 110
What Could Be the Consequences 112
What Power Do You Hold 114
Final Thoughts 116

REFERENCES 119
Images 123

PQ UNLEASHED INTRODUCTION

> *"You never touch your true potential until you challenge yourself to go beyond imposed limitations."*
>
> Roy T. Bennett

What distinguishes the average from the excellent? It's the ability to unleash the potential which lies within.

Most dictionaries define potential as the "possibility of something developing" or "something that can develop and become actual." This means that it isn't a given or automatic. Everyone has untapped potential, but potential can't grow into anything more if it isn't unleashed into action. This is what the Potential Quotient Unleashed program is here to do.

The Potential Quotient Unleashed (PQ Unleashed) program catalyzes the activation of one's potential by producing well-written books founded on research. These books aim to help readers bring out the possibilities stored within them, even and especially in specific challenging areas. Unlike other self-help books, PQ Unleashed acknowledges that one's Potential Quotient isn't fixed. It can be developed, appraised, and improved over time. Self-reflective questions are added throughout each chapter to help the reader apply various learnings, not merely based on superficial head knowledge, but through a deeper understanding of the topics' concepts.

Get ready to flourish as your potential turns into true influence and ability!

INTRODUCTION

Can you imagine putting something in your mouth and not taking note of it being there? Not realizing how the juices flow out of the center as you bite into it or how it crunches and rumbles across your teeth and tongue? If you were not able to tell how sweet it was, how much it made you squirm in sour delight, or how it simply glided down your throat, your experience of that food would be very different. It is something we do not necessarily think about and often just accept as something that ought to be. However, the taste and the enjoyment of food play a big role in our eating habits. If we did not enjoy food as much as we do, we would not be able to sustain our bodies. Enjoying the foods we eat makes us wake up and ponder what we will have for breakfast, lunch, and supper. It gives us the daily nutrition required to live life to the fullest.

Nevertheless, some of us do enjoy food a little too much. We enjoy certain types of foods more than others: foods that are very sweet, highly filling (even if we feel hungry an hour later), and foods that touch our soul. We have also come to attach a lot of meaning to the foods we enjoy. Whether that be our grandma's lasagna that brought the whole family together on Sundays; your mom's apple pie that was also considered a reward for good behavior; or the fries and ribs basket you get to share with your friends as you would share new memories and talk about old memories at the diner downtown. The stories that are entwined with the foods we eat determine how much we will love those particular foods.

We have established that eating is good for you and enjoying what you eat is even better. However, the intensity of these two elements has caused a pandemic, which has been taking the lives of millions of people each year. According to the World Health Organization (2021), "at least 2.8 million people each year die as a result of being overweight or obese." I do not know about you, but those numbers terrify me, they keep me awake at night, and they have even driven me to write this book. But, how do we control something seemingly out of our hands? There is an element of what we eat and how much we eat that the brain controls at a subconscious level. Plus, there are million-dollar companies that benefit from the status quo and can afford to keep things just as they are.

I will admit that it is not going to be easy to pull off, but it is not impossible either. There are people that have successfully done so. They eat healthily, enjoy what they eat, and lead healthy lifestyles, despite the forces acting against them. You hear them preaching their messages on your favorite podcasts, you get to catch a glimpse of their stories and tips on social media, or you might have bumped into a blog or two they have written and promoted, so when you look at them and you think that it is unimaginable to achieve. Maybe that is why you are still not eating right, still bumbling with your sugar addiction (bless those jellies), and deep down, you have given up on your capability to fight back.

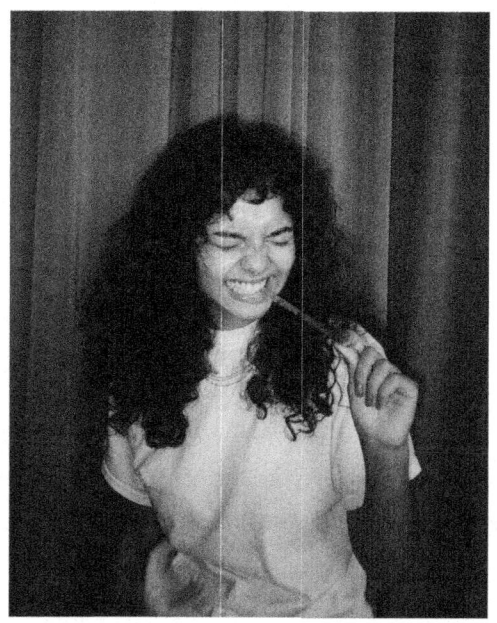

A Brief Chapter by Chapter Breakdown of the Book

Well, I am so happy you have picked up this book because I am about to show you how to fight back. This book is broken down into six core chapters. In Chapter 1, I explain exactly why you cannot seem to get enough unhealthy foods, despite the fact that you really want to. I highlight what internal and external factors keep you trapped because if you know what you are fighting against, you can put up a better fight. In the second chapter, I talk about the importance of eating healthy while enjoying your food. This is where we will break down some of the benefits of healthy eating for your body and mind. Then, in Chapter 3, we go to the opposite side of the track and highlight what will happen to your body and mind should you decide to stay on the path you are on. I will be sharing some stories about people who decided health is not a priority, not to scare you, but to motivate you to live better.

Chapter 4 covers some of the tactics health practitioners are attempting to make healthy living more appealing to you. I want you to know that you are not in this fight alone, and there are people on your side pushing you to live better. In Chapter 5, I circle back to what is preventing you from living your best, healthy life but talk more about the excuses you have been making to keep yourself trapped. If you recognize these excuses for what they really are, I believe you have a better chance of awakening yourself from that. The final chapter shares some practical steps you can implement into your daily life, enabling you to eat better and enjoy the foods that will keep your body alive. A lot of these are science-backed, so you know they will work for you. I do not want to hear anyone say: "Yes, that is great for that person, but it will not work for me."

A Book That Is Only Helpful When You Take Action

This type of thinking is what keeps you stuck in your current way of life. Break free from such thoughts, and you stand a better chance of taking the necessary actions to change your life. Remember that I can only provide you with the information; you have to apply the teachings. I do not think anyone would be reading this if they were not ready to change their lives because the information herein can be life-changing. Now, get into a quiet space, switch off your mobile phone and other distractions, get ready to take some notes or highlight key points and get ready to live the life you deserve.

CHAPTER 1

WHY WE CANNOT GET ENOUGH OF UNHEALTHY FOOD

What is your favorite food? That one thing, that no matter how terrible your day is going, you know it can pick you up. Perhaps you have more than one, and some days a donut will do, but other days, a warm serving of malva pudding drizzled with custard is the only thing that will do the trick. Why do you think you cannot stay away from these foods? Alternatively, even if you try for several days, weeks, maybe even months, then life kicks you down; you have this internal force that says: "go toward the tub of blueberry ice cream; that will magically make everything better!" Anyone that has ever been on a diet knows the feeling that overcomes your entire body when you have told yourself you would not eat sugar or any other food your diet prohibits. But then you catch yourself halfway through a bottle of soda or a packet of chips, and you are just like: "Darn it! I told myself I was not going to put this into my body, just this morning!"

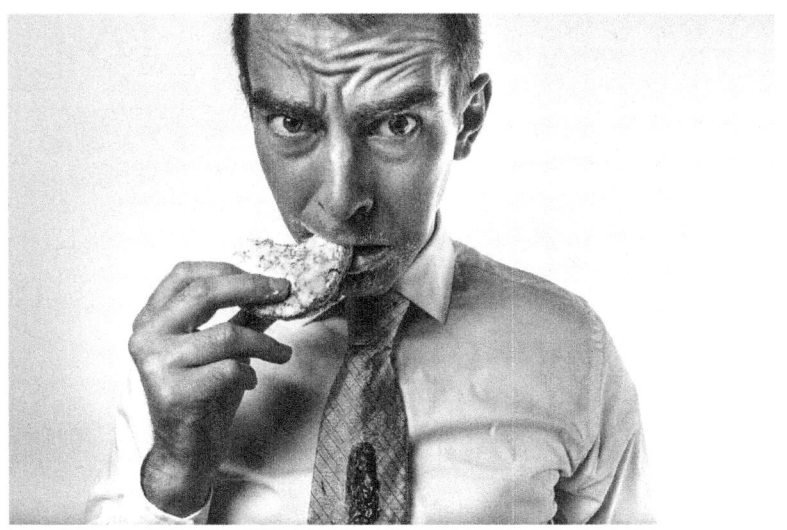

So, why cannot we stay away from foods that are considered unhealthy for us? I know you want to eat better, but something about a chocolate croissant, a cola soda, or whatever your guilty pleasure is makes staying away so tricky. The first truth is that these unhealthy foods taste so scrumptious, and a slice of carrot cake tastes much better than carrot sticks. The second truth is that we are biologically designed to seek pleasure, and stuffing your face with a triple-stacked hamburger (regardless of the consequences you will face later) is very pleasurable. This is to say, your desire and love for your favorite food, to a great extent, is not your fault. Later in the book, I will show you the means to take responsibility for what you put into your body, but for now, let us look at the things that have been driving you toward the unhealthy side of life.

The Food Industry Is Out to Take Your Money

When the industrial revolution truly boomed, agriculture and food made up a significant deal of business. For the most part, this was great: the economy grew, people obtained jobs, and more importantly, people were fed almost in abundance. Big food companies (let us not mention names) saw an opportunity to please consumers' ever-growing demands and preferences while thickening their pockets. It is not a lie; health and science reporter Kelly Crowe confirms that:

> A Google search of the patents held by the food industry provides a glimpse of the complex technical engineering that goes into building a simple cracker. Scan the scientific journals, or read the food industry publications. A picture emerges of an army of chemists, physicists, and even neuroscientists, all working to make sure you want a second cookie (Crowe, 2013).

As processed foods get created, tests are run to ensure the end result is an addictive cluster of tastes, sure to have you return for more. Meticulous attention is placed on how much sugar, salt, texture, and flavor goes into every bite. It might sound like something out of a science fiction flick, but there are actual men and women in white coats sitting in a lab, poking around with our food until it meets specific standards of taste, which over the years, they have found humans are drawn to when it comes to eating. Think about some snacks or food items that were around a decade or two ago. Maybe, the company did manage its funds poorly and ran out of business. However, it is also very likely that the foods did not live up to the human standards of what food should taste like over an extended period.

Humans are complex beings, and we like certain things in a precise way, even if we do not consciously think about them. When something does not meet our expectations anymore, we discard it (mentally and physically). These big food companies have found a way to reach deep into our unconscious preferences for food and continue to create new products that will delight our senses and have us run back to the shops ready to pay big money. Often it does not feel like a lot of money because these goods are also priced reasonably. However, those dollars add up when you calculate how much you spend on stuffing your face.

The Big Six

Think back to your favorite food: what exactly is it that you enjoy about it? Perhaps you love how its aroma can fill up an entire room. You may like the crunch or the richness in taste. Maybe you are more of a chewing fan and love how you can play around with the goods in your mouth and the flavors before you swallow the last bits. These factors, and more, are what those white-coated monsters (or geniuses) have figured out how to master when putting those foods together. According to a study put together by Witherly (2013), there are typically 16 food attributes that humans tend to look for in the foods they eat. However, only six of those are attributes that hold the highest value. A combination of these is almost always present in most of the foods we enjoy.

- **Taste hedonics:** this refers to how much salt, sugar, and umami are in the foods.

- **Dynamic contrast:** How many different flavors and textures do we enjoy from one item?

- **Evoked qualities:** the foods themselves remind us of past experiences.

- **The food pleasure equation:** Macronutrients (carbs, protein, fats) + Sensation (texture, aroma, taste) = Food pleasure.

- **Caloric density:** How many calories and energy is available within the goods per serving size? We do not want to feel like it is too high (even when it is).

- **Emulsion Theory:** Foods have to be salty and fatty or sugary and fatty (and, if possible, all three simultaneously).

I am sure you are salivating right now (another one of the 16 attributes) just thinking about your favorite foods. You can see how they fit into these six factors. They were designed to be just like that. They were intended to taste incredibly good, more than fresh fruits and vegetables from the soil. These companies knew that processing food in this particular manner would have us coming back for more, reaching deeper into our pockets, and ultimately eating ourselves to death: they even have products called "death by chocolate!" Okay, this last part is an exaggeration, not the product name—that is a real thing, but the part where they intended for these products to kill us.

According to the article by Kelly Crowe (2013), a lot of these scientists and food engineers, upon more and more cases of poor health showing up, have decided to hang up their white coats because they could not handle being at the source of death to millions of people. Others have decided to take their skills and process healthier alternatives (more on this later). Most of them continue to hang their heads low and do what they are being paid to do. There is someone that is going to have to do that job, right? Now, before we go off topic here, let us slide back to the big six and break them down further.

Taste Hedonics

Taste is an essential sensory experience for humans. From an evolutionary point of view, our predecessors did not have food packaged in boxes with a smiley face on it to tell them whether something was good or not. They had to test some foods themselves. If something tastes good, they immediately assign a "safe" label to it. That label gets taught to others in the tribe and future generations after that. Today, we are spoiled for choice, we already have an abundance of natural food that we know is safe for us, but I supposed that was not enough for us. Our intelligent little brains had to find something better, which they did. However, even with processed foods, there are a million options, so big food brands have to ensure that their products taste better than anything else you will ever get your hands on.

Taste essentially comes down to sugar, salt, fats, as well as what is referred to as umami. According to health blogger Ryan Raman (2019), umami is considered the fifth taste sensation alongside sweet, salty, sour, and bitter. The term is Japanese, and it stands for deliciousness. However, it can roughly be translated into a savory sense or even meaty taste. A rich pot of beef stew or even a piece of pork ribs would not be considered sweet or necessarily salty, but rather umami. Now, I wanted to highlight this taste sensation more than the others here because umami refers to the taste of glutamate, an amino acid found in vegetable and animal proteins. Although it can be found naturally in many common processed foods, the people in the white coats had to create something called monosodium glutamate (MSG) to duplicate that sense of deliciousness that is so important to our taste buds.

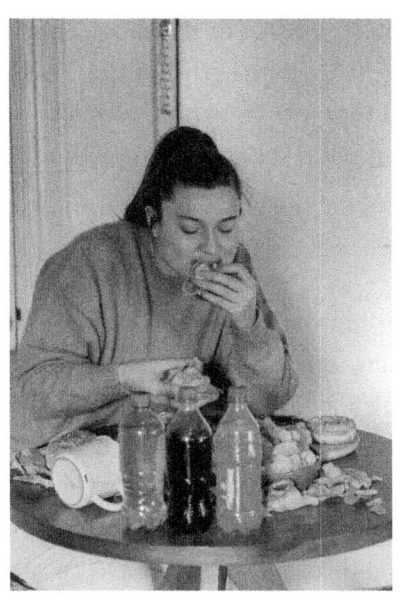

Anyone reading this book that's even remotely health-conscious should have heard this term being thrown around a lot, essentially the message coming down to "if you see this product in your foods, run away." Rightly so, and I will discuss some reasons for this in Chapter 3. The point I am trying to make here is that big food brands have even gone as far as manufacturing a taste so we can enjoy their products more. They even know how much of these taste factors need to go into a particular product for it to be considered *yummy*. For example, the percentage of salt should always be between 1.0 and 1.5. But the taste, according to Witherly (2013), only makes up 10% of what we enjoy about our favorite foods. The other five attributes (as well as the other 15) also play a massive role in how we view and get to enjoy the foods we eat.

Dynamic Contrast

There are two components to this: the physical taste of the goods is vital, but their appearance here is also essential. The more textures and flavors a single product has, the more we enjoy it. Think about a crunchy bar of chocolate: smooth, crunchy, and gooey. Plus, it is sweet and salty. Why do you think big food brands play around with so many flavors and designs and even add artificial flavors to these products, giving off the impression of a flavor that's not even there? Add a dash, no, a splash of color to the mix, and our eyes and tummies get hungrier. Humans are highly visual creatures. We experience a lot with our eyes alone. If something looks good, we instantly assume it tastes good (perhaps even makes us believe it *has* to taste good).

A lot of money goes into packaging alone. "Typically, companies spend 10-40% of the product's retail price on the packaging. For example, if the product sells $100, then the company might spend anywhere between $10-$40 on the packaging" (Madhurakavi, 2021). I can almost guarantee you that the ones that spend more on the packaging, in terms of both time and money, sell more products.

Brighter colors, a fun shape, large fonts on the stuff that matters (like Super Yummy), and small fonts on the things that will catch them out (like product ingredients). We tend to focus on what we can see first and most outwardly. No one really has time to turn the box over, let alone research what sodium nitrite actually means. If you were waiting for the answer, I would not give it to you. Go research it; this is the perfect time to get some practice.

Evoked Qualities

Humans learn through the recognition of patterns. We also love new experiences but still want a sense of familiarity. This is achieved in food through a subtle blend of familiar flavors. This is why corn chips, for example, tend to use familiar foods such as flavors like cheese, salt, vinegar, BBQ, tomato, etcetera. These flavors and foods remind us of other pleasing foods (and even experiences like a BBQ with family and friends). In addition, there has been a trend in recent years to include an entire meal from a particular country and cultural group to further evoke feelings of familiarity with the products. People from those cultures want to experience their favorite childhood meal as a snack, and people from other cultures are curious to find out what other people eat.

Some brands with a lot of money will also evoke some experiences as part of their marketing campaigns. For example, the idea of a particular snack bringing people together, making them stand out and be unique, or being the source of love is constantly being shared through advertising and media outlets. Seeing other people like you, or who seem to enjoy the life you want to have, somehow makes you feel like you should too be eating those foods as portrayed in the ads. This process can happen instantly or over a couple of months through re-exposure. For example, suppose you see an advertisement about a particular product all the time. In that case, you eventually decide you must try it (anyone willing to spend so much money on something must have something good to offer, right?) So, you give it a shot, and next thing you know, you feel like that person in the ad, and like that feeling, so you keep buying those goods.

The Food Pleasure Equation

As mentioned, our overall experience of pleasure from the foods we eat is made up of a combination of the macronutrients and the sense experience, or dynamism, of the foods. Think about a warm bowl of meatballs and pasta. Proteins from the mincemeat, carbohydrates from the linguine, and fats (some of which are healthy) from the cheese and perhaps other sauces added to the dish make this a macronutrient-dense meal with a lot of different flavors and textures to chew through and slurp up. There is no question why many people love this meal and similar meals.

Not all three of these macronutrients have to be available at once, and sometimes two can be prominent. At the same time, it just adds more of a punch if all three are there, like with a creamy, sweet, and tangy cheesecake. Nevertheless, what matters is that both macronutrients and a powerful sensory experience are present. Witherly explains that foods are not rich in macronutrients; they have to make up for this through the sensory experience like chunky and crunchy corn chips or chewy and gooey jelly candy. Plus, these still get their good filling of salt, sugar, fats, and artificial umami. The same goes for low-fat products (usually dairy products); these get packed with more sugar to compensate for the loss of the fatty macronutrient.

Caloric Density

Caloric density is evaluated as a score between 0 and 9. Water would have a score of 0, and pure fat would score 9. The mind and body consider a "good score" to be a caloric density of between 4 and 5, which is how most processed foods are designed to be scored. I said mind and body intentionally—there is a neural connection between your gut and brain (referred to as the gut-brain axis or GBA). Your gut sends information to your brain on everything you have just eaten, and the brain interprets these messages almost instantly. This is also why foods that are not high in calories and are not considered delectable, like a bowl of kale or even a ripe red tomato, automatically gets registered as "not so enjoyable." We do not necessarily want to eat more of them.

Your eyes, mouth, gut, and brain work collaboratively to tell you when you are supposed to be satiated. You dish up a big plate of food, you munch through all of it, your GBA senses you have had a caloric dense meal of 4.5, and so you gobble down a glass of soda and say: "Yes, I have had a full lunch, I am full now." However, this does not happen with some foods, like popcorn, ice cream, pretzel sticks, twists, or even soda. Although these products have a high caloric density, they seem to melt away in your mouth before the GBA has enough time to establish how much you have consumed through your mouth. Nothing or not much passed through the teeth long enough for that connection to be made. That is why you can sit through a 90-minute movie, put handful after handful of popcorn in your mouth, slurp down your XL soda, and still leave the theater ready to have dinner or lunch.

Emulsion Theory

An emulsion of food is typically a combination of different foods and tastes into one so that the result is a creation of a more robust taste. Ice cream, for example, is an emulsion, where milk (which is high in fats), sweeteners, and other solids (like fruit chunks or chocolate) get combined to form a frozen emulsion. However, the sugars are concentrated through this process, making the final product even sweeter. Have you ever noticed how you can quickly overdo the salt when making mashed potatoes? Witherly explains that the salt content in butter alone is about 2.5%. However, when emulsified with other ingredients like potatoes, crème, or milk, it increases to 10%. This piece of information was such a lifesaver to my mid-week mash.

Now, the men and women in the white coats can bring out certain flavors in the foods because they use this theory. Ice cream, ready-to-eat cottage pie, chocolate, and some of our favorite sauces are all examples of emulsions that have been carefully formulated and designed to be irresistible and make you want just a little more, which never ends up being a small amount. Combine this factor with some of the points discussed earlier on taste and dynamic contrast, and it is no surprise you have not been able to escape your current unhealthy lifestyle.

The Bliss Point

Big food and beverage companies spend a lot of money hiring researchers, scientists, and brain specialists to ensure that when their products enter through your lips, you experience what is known as "the bliss point" (Crowe, 2013). They make that money back 10-fold, so do not feel bad for them. By taking the time to get the salt, sugar, fats, and artificial umami measurements just right, they are able to create something that will lure you mentally and physically to come back for more, to spend more. Processed foods without these additives would be unbearable, and I am not exaggerating to make a point. One of the journalists Crowe was working with was invited to some of these big food companies to get a taste tour.

He explained that cereal without sugar tasted like metal, and crackers without salt were not swallowable. It is not real food, people. Despite how they position it and all the added "vitamins" or nutritional factors they may add to some of their goods, the fact is, processed foods would not qualify as food if it were not for the added flavors (natural and artificial). Their purpose is not to keep us satiated with the right combination of nutrients. Some of the men and women in the white coats have admitted that "the most highly loaded salty, sugary, fatty foods are every bit as addictive as some narcotics" (Crowe, 2013). So, their purpose is to keep us craving for more, and like with any other craving when it hits, there is this internal driving force that says you have to get your fix. Ultimately, after all the years of overeating, diabetes, high blood pressure, obesity, and heart disease, the consumer is not the one who will be experiencing bliss.

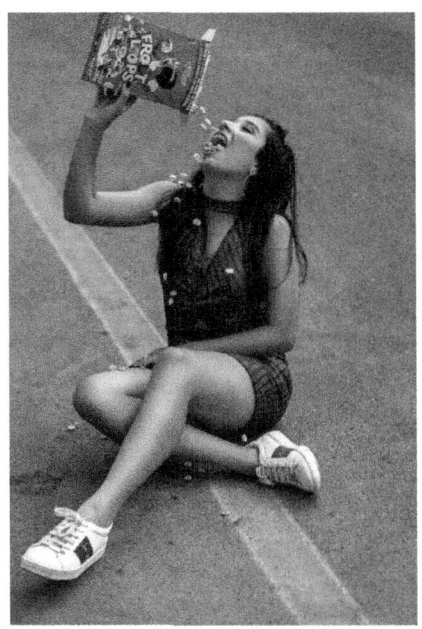

Your Food Addiction and Dopamine

Your brain has an internal mechanism designed to motivate you to seek things that will bring you pleasure. We can all agree that food brings us pleasure. Initially (I am talking hunter-gatherer times now), the idea was that when we feel hungry, we get up and look for what we have to eat, we feel happy about the hunt, we feel so glad about the food, and we would find something else to keep our minds busy. Now, that initial feeling of excitement to hunt for food is caused by a minor release of dopamine in the brain. When we get what we want, in this case, a good piece of meat, more dopamine is released, making us feel even more pleasure. Welcome evolution and human advancements; now, we do not even have to hunt for our food; it gets delivered to our doorstep. But now, the steak comes basted in so many sauces and flavors that the amount of dopamine released is even higher than in ancient times, which is not good.

So, what exactly is dopamine, and why would something that makes us feel good becomes bad for us in high quantities? According to an article published in *Cleveland Clinic* (2022), dopamine is a neurotransmitter in the brain that "plays a role as a "reward center" and in many body functions, including memory, movement, motivation, mood, attention and more." The more dopamine a particular activity releases, the more we want to participate in it. However, your brain can release only so much dopamine at any specific time, so doing more of that activity does not make you happier. Plus, after you have experienced the high levels of dopamine, your brain tries to reset itself by making you experience an equal amount of "sadness" in relation to how happy you have been.

I will be using arbitrary numbers here, but let us say your average level of dopamine is about 5. You eat a piece of chocolate (which has been shown to increase your dopamine levels by up to 150%), and your dopamine levels spike to 7.5. As dopamine levels decrease, they do not come back to 5 but rather to about 2.5. So, you feel unhappier than before you ate the chocolate. Naturally, the brain will bring itself back up to 5. However, most people have an unconscious panic, thinking they have to eat more chocolate to feel better. Plus, it tastes so good, so you do not get full, and you end up eating more than necessary in hopes of getting your happiness levels back up, which never happens.

What is even scarier is that the more you do the activity (in this case, eat), the more difficult it will be to get happier from the same thing.

After a while, your brain grows a sort of tolerance so that it can feel like even the creamiest ice cream does not make you happy anymore. However, because you remember a time when it did, you still continue eating more of it, and it still tastes reasonably good as it was designed. Now, you are stuck with the problem of eating more, but you are not necessarily even getting happy by doing so. It is a sad vicious cycle that many overweight and obese people struggle with throughout their lives. Interestingly, the Cleveland Clinic article also mentions that people with high dopamine levels are more likely to develop addictions and become obese. This is because they have a higher drive to do the things that would make them feel happy even when everything else in their lives says stop.

Another problem with the release of dopamine and food addictions is that we get to want more of those foods that release the most pleasure, like processed foods that are high in sugar, salt, fats, and artificial additives. To the extent that "normal" food tastes particularly terrible. We can no longer appreciate healthy foods like broccoli or corn (unless they are garnished in creams, butter, and sauces), making healthy eating a significant obstacle. We would rather opt for fries than baked potatoes because the former is dunked into unhealthy fats and can be lathered in all types of yummy sauces. We have lost our taste for the foods that can sustain our bodies and have been sustaining us for the past centuries. So again, if you have been struggling to be healthy, eat and live well, it is not entirely on you. Your brain and the environment you are in have made this task especially difficult for you. But, now that you are aware of these mental and physical barriers, you can work around them.

Key Takeaways

- Regardless of how hard they try, many people are drawn to unhealthy foods that are highly processed and provide little nutritional value. This is because there are people with more money and power pulling the strings, putting together food creations designed to keep you addicted.

- There are approximately 16 food attributes big food, and beverage companies play around with to create products that excite your mouth and brain, luring you back for one more bite. The top six attributes are taste hedonics, dynamic contrast, evoked qualities, the food pleasure equation, caloric density, and emulsion theory.

- At a distance, these food attributes seem like they are harmless. However, upon closer scrutiny, you would find that they are used only to mask the sinister smells, tastes, and textures processed foods harbor. This is done all in an effort to keep consumers addicted, hungry for more, and willing to pay any price to acquire more.

- Food addiction is real and is every bit as self-destroying as a narcotic. Foods that taste great and are made with just the right combinations of sugar, salt, and fat release a significant amount of dopamine, the hormone associated with pleasure. Once the dopamine drops, you try to get that feeling of bliss back by eating more of those products. Suppose you want to break free from your food addiction. In that case, you first have to ask yourself if the taste quality of these products, which can be essentially poisonous, is worth your well-being.

CHAPTER 2

THE IMPORTANCE OF EATING HEALTHY AND ENJOYING YOUR FOOD

What is your favorite vegetable or fruit? Some people might hate all types of vegetables, but there is no way you could also hate all fruits. Perhaps you do not enjoy them as much as you would crunching on some chips, but there are some that you enjoy or at least tolerate. Anytime we enjoy something, we want more of it due to dopamine. However, this is not only something that happens to us passively; we have a choice in doing it. You choose to like pears instead of apples. You decide to grab grapes instead of strawberries. Even with unhealthy foods, some people prefer cookies, which would not please another person who loves to eat burgers, sausages, and bacon. Consequently, the amount of dopamine released after eating a particular product also comes down to preference and choice—there is no universal law to it.

Even as it pertains to activities, not just food, for example, someone that enjoys exercise can experience an increase in dopamine levels up to 200% after a good workout. But for someone who hates working out, no pleasurable feelings and hormones will be released. Again, whether or not you enjoy exercise comes down to a choice. So, you can choose to live a healthy lifestyle, and you can choose to enjoy healthy foods. This latter point is critical because if you do not enjoy something, or you do not tell your mind that you enjoy a particular thing, you will automatically move away from it. Remember, our brains are designed to seek pleasure. Nevertheless, it is not that all things are intrinsically pleasurable; we get to decide what we enjoy and do not have to care much for food.

Previously, you have decided that eating healthy foods is not delicious, or at least not as tasty as unhealthy foods, or just processed foods in general. This choice is something that can easily be reversed. According to neuroscientist Andrew Huberman (2021), due to the release of dopamine:

> Those highly palatable foods are making more bland foods, more whole foods, meaning foods that are not processed… taste less good, at least for a while. Moreover, all it takes is a short period of time, even just days, two days or so of not consuming any highly palatable foods, and suddenly broccoli with just a little bit of seasoning tastes delicious to you.

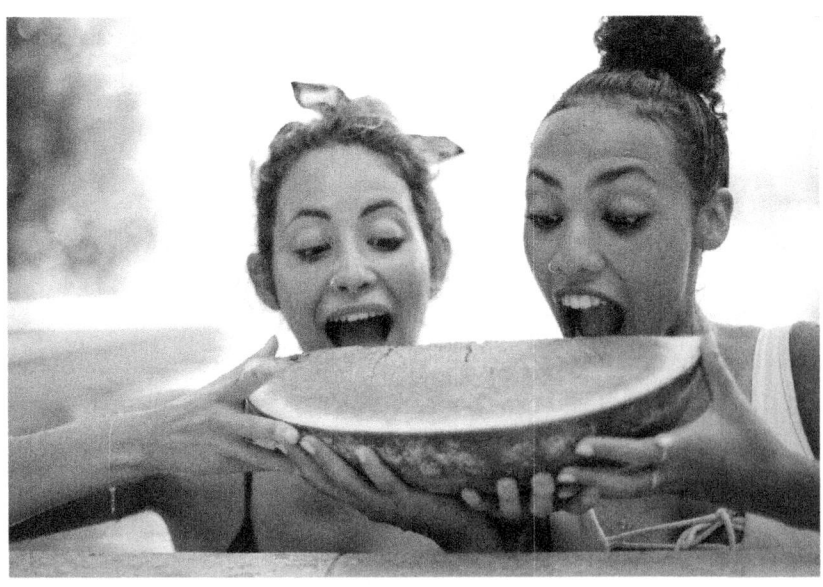

Suppose you are someone that has been eating poorly for several decades now. For instance, there are no home-cooked meals, high-sugar breakfast, fatty takeaways for lunch and supper, and constant snacking between meals. This will no doubt be a more significant challenge to you and may take longer to overcome than for someone who has tried to squeeze in a few healthy eating habits now and again. However, it is possible for any person; your brain is capable of taking on new routines and habits.

Why You Should Eat Healthily

Do not get too caught up in specific diets, eating plans, or nutritional rules like counting calories. Instead, you want to focus on cutting back on foods high in sugar, salt, and unhealthy fats. Whether you are a vegetarian, following the Paleo diet, or practicing intermittent fasting is not as crucial as deciding that you are going to choose whole foods over processed foods full-time or at least 80% of the time. According to Franziska Spritzler (2021), a dietician and diabetes educator, whole foods are free from chemical additives, do not get formulated in a factory, and come packed with macronutrients. This should be enough to make anyone leave the dark side for good. But in case you are not convinced yet, here are some additional benefits of choosing to be healthy:

- **Chances of overeating are minimum:** Whole foods are not as addictive as processed foods, so the chances of your mind craving more are not likely. Overeating on grapes or cucumber sticks will not have as many adverse side effects as eating a whole tub of ice cream.

- **Good for your gut health:** Because of the gut-brain axis (GBA), anything that promotes a healthy gut ultimately stimulates a healthy brain. So, with healthy eating, you boost your brain's power, enabling you to perform better in life.

- **Suitable for the heart:** Whole foods lower inflammation and contain antioxidants that promote heart health, lowering your chances of suffering from heart disease or other heart-related issues.

- **Low in sugar and salt:** Most whole foods contain natural amounts of sugar and salt. These are not high enough to get you addicted and come packed with other nutritional sources like vitamins, water, or fiber, making them excellent alternatives to processed foods.

- **High in fiber:** Fiber is excellent for gut health and your entire digestive system. Eating foods high in fiber also makes you feel satiated for longer, making you less likely to crave snacks between meals.

- **High in healthy fats:** The term fats have previously been frowned upon, especially with the idea that fats are what cause people to gain weight. Although this is partially true, recent studies have shown that only unhealthy fats (for example, trans fats) promote weight gain. Whereas healthy fats (like unsaturated fats) can promote weight loss when incorporated into the right diet and eating plan. Healthy fats also promote heart health.

- **Reduces your risk of disease:** It has been shown that healthy eating is directly correlated to lower chances of getting heart disease, diabetes, cancer, metabolic syndrome, and obesity, just to name a few.

- **Better dental health:** Foods high in sugar are corrosive to dental health and promote cavities and plaque buildup. Healthy foods like cheese and green tea, on the other hand, have been shown to protect tooth enamel and prevent cavities.

- **Promotes better skin:** Whole foods help nourish and protect your skin, as does drinking lots of water (instead of sugary beverages). Whole foods protect against acne, reduce wrinkling and promote elasticity, especially as you age. Processed foods promote the appearance and severity of acne.

- **It costs less in the long run:** It has been shown that people who eat healthily spend more money on food than those who eat processed foods. However, it is also the case that people who eat unhealthy foods are more likely to fall ill. So, paying to control a disease like diabetes is more costly than any diet.

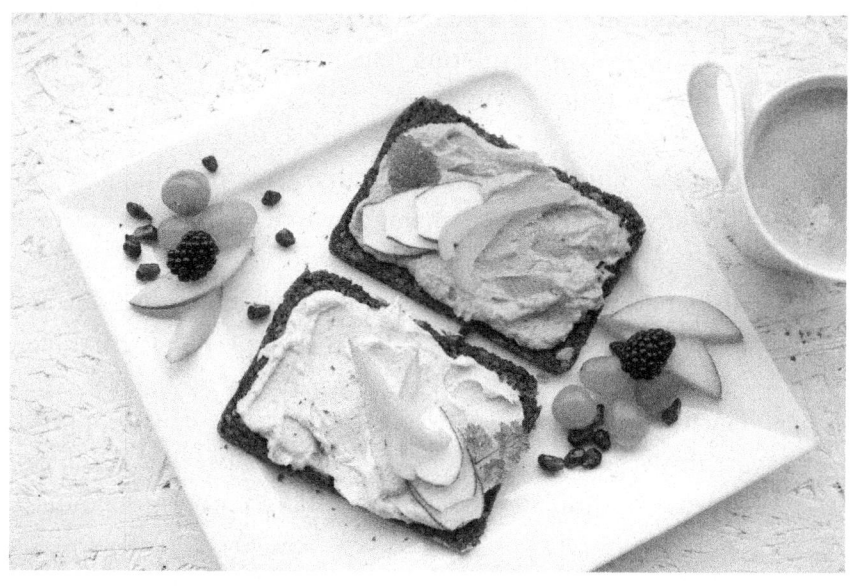

Tips to Make Your Food Taste Better

You have to enjoy the food you eat, but you do not have to buy fast food or processed goods off a grocery shelf in order for you to receive the deliciousness of food. Cooking your own meals will almost always be healthier than buying ready-to-eat products. Making your own burger patties from compressed beef mince, seasoned well and brought together with some egg yolk, then added to your bun with the typical garnishes will be healthier than any burger you order from a takeaway joint. Top that up with baked potatoes instead of fries and some freshly squeezed orange juice rather than a soda, and you will very well qualify for "Health Nut of the Year." All it takes for you to enjoy healthy eating is to choose to stay away from processed foods and pay special attention to how you cook your food and what you add to it. According to Witherly (2013), there are some healthy foods and add-ons which can make any meal taste like you are fresh out of culinary school, such as:

- **Soy Sauce.** Opt for an MSG-free version, and you will have access to a flavorful mixture that works well with both savory and sweet dishes.

- **Cheese.** This is high in healthy fats, protein, and flavor-active compounds, making many foods taste creamier and more decadent, especially savory dishes. Use cheddar, Romano, and parmesan, as not all cheeses are healthy, and not all of them blend well with other foods like these three.

- **Garlic.** Not everyone loves garlic, but those who appreciate this vegetable's rich aroma. Garlic is especially significant because it stimulates the umami taste receptor in the mouth.

- **Butter.** This water-in-oil emulsion contains flavor-boosting glutamates that make anything taste much better. Plus, butter has high dynamic contrast as it feels like it melts away in your mouth upon consumption.

- **Shallots.** These are an excellent replacement for onions, as they bring out all the flavor in foods without the lingering taste of the vegetable like you would find with onions. It is also high in sugar, allowing it to caramelize faster even in low heat.

- **Sugar.** In small quantities, sugar is good in food. Replacing white sugar with brown sugar, maple syrup, or honey can also be healthier. You can also add these to both sweet and savory dishes, enhancing the hedonic element of your food without any repercussions.

- **Worcestershire Sauce.** Do not worry about the pronunciation; this is a concoction that can be used to add volume to sauces and light flavor to the meat. Frequently used as a replacement for soy sauce, but it has more additives like vinegar, corn syrup, molasses, onions, garlic, chili pepper extract, and a few more.

- **Bacon.** You see, we are not cutting out all the good stuff. Good-quality bacon is high in nutrients and flavorings that make most dishes (especially your vegetables) taste amazing.

- **Egg Yolks.** You may be surprised to find that many of your favorite food emulsions contain egg yolks. Egg yolks are great because they are high in nutrients (particularly protein and fats) and vitamins (like A, D, E, and K), yet they make food taste good. As mentioned, you can add them to homemade patties, but also sauces and some desserts.

- **Salts, spices, and herbs.** Salt, in reasonable quantities, is necessary for food to be edible and does have some health benefits for you (improves sleep, supports the nervous system, supports hydration). Try using fresh herbs instead of dried versions (especially for parsley and basil), as the taste and benefits are not the same. Finally, do not be afraid to blend different spices instead of using only one or two per meal. You can create your own formulations or buy them ready-blended.

A 10-Day Detox Diet Plan

Ten days without any snacks, heavily processed foods, or no desserts may seem like a living hell at this moment, but those days will fly by before you know it. The purpose of the detox is to reset the taste receptors in your mouth and brain so you can enjoy healthy, home-cooked meals made with vegetables and to view a handful of sweet green grapes as a viable snack option. Make full use of that list of flavorful additives, which brings out the best in almost every meal. This is the best time for you to explore flavors but always do additional research into what will work best and what just will not. The last thing you need is for this experiment to garner poor taste, as that is the opposite of what is intended here.

For the next ten days, you will exclusively eat whole foods. If you want to subscribe to a particular diet, you can do so. To make things easier, I will provide you with some hearty meal options. These are some of my tried and tested recipes, so I know you will enjoy them. However, feel free to change some of the ingredients as you see fit. Do not forget to drink lots of water during the detox. Water helps you feel satiated and enables you to get rid of unwanted bodily toxins. Do not beat yourself up if you accidentally grab and eat something unhealthy. Having a snack because we are bored or because we have made ourselves believe it helps us focus better is a bad habit that can take several months for some people to shake.

Take note of what typically triggers you to want to eat unhealthy foods and snacks. If you find you have a snack when you are watching television, actively remind yourself that you do not need to eat every time you sit down to watch your favorite TV show. If you feel like you have to munch on something, grab a handful of cashews, walnuts, or a mixture of both. Some people are stress-eaters and are drawn to junk food due to circumstances at work or home. Learning to process stress in healthier ways (talking, taking a walk, or going for a back massage) can help ease the pressure from stress. Again, find a healthy habit or snack to replace the bad. So, if you usually chew on jelly-like candy when you are stressed, you can choose to make or buy a fruit salad. After all, those candies are said to be fruit-flavored, so why not enjoy the real thing?

What Are You Going to Eat?

On day one, start your morning with some eggs, tomatoes (cocktail tomatoes work best because they are sweet and small), and cheese muffins. These are simple to make and go well with orange juice, a glass of milk, or your traditional morning coffee if you do not function without caffeine. In the afternoon, make yourself a homemade burger and a side salad. For dinner, you can enjoy beef stew (add three to four vegetables like carrots, marrow, potatoes, corn, butternut cubes, or even beans) with brown rice or quinoa. White rice is more processed, so it loses some of its nutrients by the time it reaches the store. If you can, make a larger batch of food than what you need on the day; this way, you do not have to cook every day, all week. This is one of the reasons why people opt to buy takeaways; they are more convenient on those days when you are lazy or busy.

On the second day, if you made extra muffins (most recipes will have you make 12, and you can store them in the fridge or freezer), have them for breakfast. At lunch, you can have some leftover stew. In the evening, make yourself a fresh green salad and chicken breast. For the salad, I always drizzle over a concoction of olive oil, lemon, and honey, with some salt and pepper. Store-bought salad dressings can come with more sugar and salt than necessary, defeating the whole purpose of the salad.

You can switch up your morning on day three with a fruit salad by mixing chopped apples, grapes, oranges, kiwi fruit, bananas, and pineapples (or any of your favorite fruit) in a cereal bowl. You can add plain yogurt and some honey for extra flavor, but these are not essential. Lunchtime will have you enjoying chicken (leftover chicken breast) and mayo toasties. You do not have to toast your bread, but some people prefer it that way. I suggest you go for brown or whole-wheat, instead of white bread. For supper, if you still have leftover chicken, have a piece with a bit of rice (a serving about the size of your palm), with honey-glazed carrots and cheesy broccoli.

Day four can be started with another fruit salad, or you can turn your ingredients into a smoothie. If you are not a fan of cow's milk, coconut or almond milk can do the trick, but I prefer the taste of the former option. For lunch, you can have eggs, cheese, and tomato toasties, and if you like, toss in some bacon. You might still have some carrots left at dinner, but if you do not, they are quick and easy to make, so do so. Make a side serving of spinach as well, you can make it creamy with cream and cheese, or you can have it savory with garlic and butter. For protein, you can enjoy a hake filet, tenderized steak, or pork chop—each of these is quick to make and can be pan-fried for your convenience.

Start your day five with eggs, cheese, and spinach muffins. These taste better than they sound and can taste even better with some bacon pieces. In the afternoon, have a salad, and toss some leftover meat all over it. Drizzle with your homemade dressing, and enjoy. For dinner, indulge yourself in a cottage pie. For the Mash potato topping, do not forget to add sour cream or Fromage Frais/Blanc to add an extra layer of creamy flavor. You can add any combination of vegetables to your beef mince for the filling. Some great options are carrots, celery, butternut, carrots, peas, and sweet corn. Do not forget to add a mixture of spices, herbs, and your favorite sweetener; you have to use garlic. For the sauce, you can use beef stock, soy sauce, Worcestershire sauce, balsamic vinegar, and tomato puree. Feel free to play around with other alternatives, and enjoy.

On the sixth day, you can wake up to some leftover muffins. Leftover cottage pie will be for lunch or supper, and the third meal of the day can be something light like a salad, a sandwich, or a bowl of roasted vegetables. The option you go with should not be calorie-dense. It should be just filling enough that you will not feel hungry within the next hour or so or have to wake up in the middle of the night to grab whatever you can find in the fridge. If you feel hungry, grab a fruit and drink some water, which usually does the trick.

The seventh day would be the perfect time to switch up your breakfast with a warm bowl of oats. Add milk, butter, bananas (or berries), honey, and a pinch of salt, for a filling breakfast that is flavorful and has some dynamic contrast. For lunch, try something different like a chicken wrap, but instead of bread or a tortilla, you wrap it up in leaves of lettuce. When supper time comes around, make some chicken breast and two vegetables. Try to change it up from the meal on day three. So, if you made the chicken breast in the oven last time, you can now sear it in a pan. For the vegetables, try some sweet potatoes (mashed or baked wedges can be great options) and green beans with garlic and cocktail tomatoes.

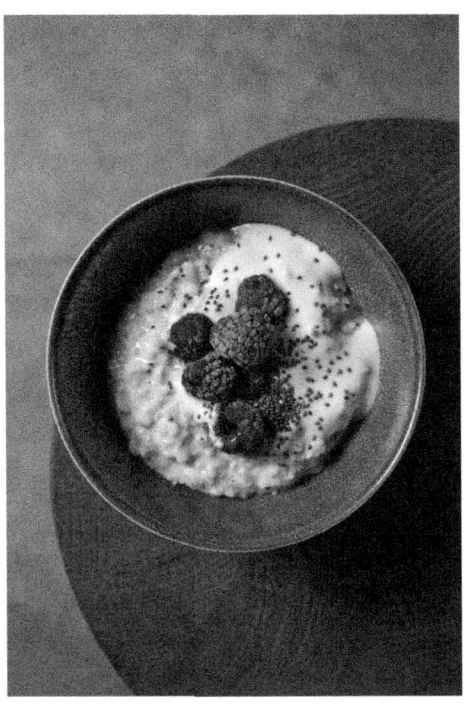

The morning of day eight can start with another bowl of oats. If you tried the ingredients mentioned above, you would want to have this every day. In the afternoon, make a tuna and cheese melt. You can always make it with leftover chicken breast if you have found you made enough. However, tuna has this melt-in-mouth effect that no other source can bring. End your day with a bowl of fusilli pasta and lamb ragu. This is an Italian-inspired dish made from pasta, boneless lamb pieces, peeled tomatoes or tomato puree, red wine, and Romano cheese to drizzle over the top. Your garlic, spices, and herbs are still a yes. Although most people enjoy this meal as is, and chances are you will too, you can add olives or mushrooms to the mixture. Any additive that cooks quickly and has a subtle taste will work well here.

On day nine, enjoy a big English breakfast of fried eggs, baked beans, tomatoes, mushrooms, bacon, sausages, and toast. Hopefully, you did not get to add all the fusilli to the lamb sauce last night; you can use it to make a bowl of pasta salad for lunch. For your own reference, this goes well as a dish on its own but can also be used as a side to the main dish. When dinner comes around, pop some bone-in chicken pieces and mixed vegetable chunks (like potatoes, carrots, butternut, and zucchini) into the oven, covered in various herbs and spices.

Enjoy a fruit bowl in the morning on your detox's final day. Switch up the fruits from last time. For lunch, have a classic bacon and egg sandwich. Finally, end your detox with some leftover chicken and baked vegetables. By now, you should have gained your love for simple good food back and even considered making this your new lifestyle. You should seriously consider this, and I will show you why in the next chapter.

Working Around the Obstacles

I know some of you might be thinking that this looks all good and well, but you are already giving yourself a reason to back out. Perhaps you do not have enough time. Some of you work long hours, and cooking a three-hour stew might not fit your schedule. Surely you have some time off. Use your time off to cook some meals in advance, or if you can afford to, pay someone to cook your meals for these ten days until you can recognize the goodness of eating healthy and want to do this for yourself continuously. Some of you might be worried that you will not be able to have leftovers like in the examples given above because you have to cook for a family of four, six, or maybe even more. You will be required to cook more often in this case. You can ask your family to get involved in cooking meals. This way, you do not have to do it all yourself, and you get to bond over making dinner.

Key Takeaways

- If there were ever a better time to stay away from sugar, salt, and unhealthy fats, that time would be long gone. The next best time is now. Eating healthy has a wide range of benefits that go beyond manufactured taste. Healthy foods make you feel fuller for longer; support gut, heart, and dental health; reduce your risk of disease; are low in salt and sugar but high in fiber and good fats; make you look and feel good; will not cost you your life.

- Unfortunately, the taste still plays a significant role in our eating choices. So, if you want to make healthy eating your preferred choice, you have to cook your meals in such a way that it encourages this food attribute. Some foods and nutritional additives that can make your meals taste excellent include soy sauce, cheese, garlic, butter, shallots, sugar, Worcestershire sauce, bacon, egg yolks, and a range of fresh herbs and spices.

- Stay away from unhealthy foods for at least ten days to bring back your love for healthy foods. During this period, you are only allowed to eat whole foods, ensuring you stay away from processed foods and beverages. This time away from unhealthy foods will give you time to reset your taste receptors. You might also become more aware of the foods that work well for your body versus those that are not so aligned (even though they are healthy. After all, everybody is different and has different nutritional needs.

- Ask yourself, are you not willing to sacrifice ten days of your life to get back ten years? This little experiment can set the trajectory of the rest of your life. Failure to act at this point would result in some profound health implications.

CHAPTER 3

THE CONSEQUENCES OF NOT LEADING A HEALTHY LIFESTYLE

When you hear the words "good food," what comes to mind should not just be foods that taste good, but foods that are good for your body and will contribute to you living a quality life. You need to value the quality of your life more than your tongue. If you do not, bad, bad things are going to happen to you. I am being serious here; when you do not eat healthily, you put your body and mind at risk of developing diseases. For the longest time, medical science was not sure what to do about illnesses such as autoimmune diseases. It was not certain how they came about. What is known, however, is that highly processed foods became popular around the 19th century, and "medical historians identify the mid-20th century as the time when the scientific and medical communities acknowledged the existence of autoimmune disease" (Margo & Harman, 2016).

According to Singh et al. (2016), autoimmune diseases refer to "pathological conditions identified by abnormal autoimmune responses and characterized by auto-antibodies and T-cell responses to self-molecules by immune system reactivity." What happens is that the body does not recognize which cells and microorganisms belong to it versus foreign objects that need demolishing. So, it attacks both, resulting in damage to its own cells, causing the amplification of that disease. Whatever you eat gets processed through the digestive system; the body takes the needed molecules and discards what is not. Processed foods are meant to mimic natural foods in taste and function, but they are not real.

The body digests some of the foreign particles that make up a large volume of processed foods; it later realizes that there is something not exactly right. It tries to fight off these foreign bodies. However, it cannot distinguish where the human cells begin and the end of the foreign cells, so everything gets attacked, hoping it will get some of the bad stuff out. We know this does not occur; instead, we find diseases such as rheumatoid arthritis, type 2 diabetes, and lupus. More men and women in white coats come together and try to create medicine to manage these diseases. They do an average job (some like Moynihan et al. (2002) and Rang (2013) might speculate, intentionally) at managing these diseases. However, they continue feeding off gullible and desperate people who are experiencing real pain.

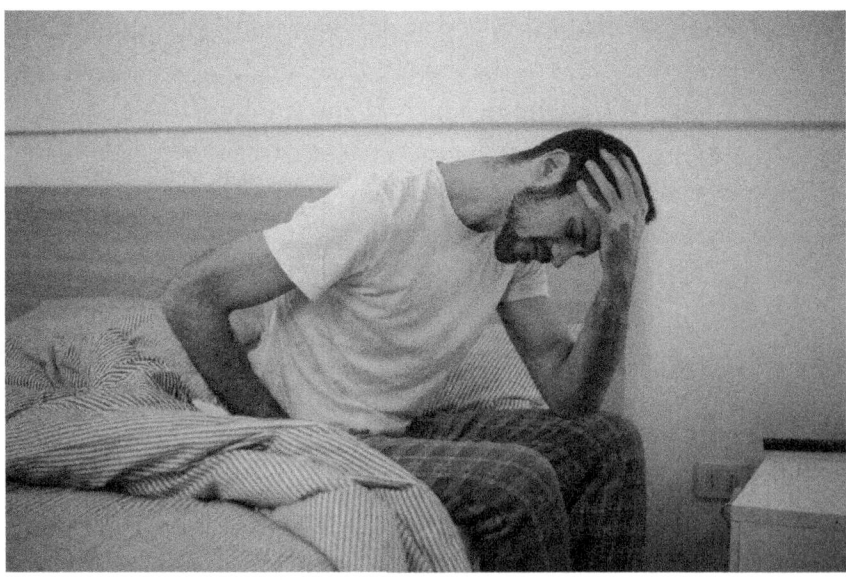

The intention of this book is not to call out big food or pharmaceutical companies but to slightly open your eyes to what is happening worldwide. If you can see what you are buying into, you can make more informed decisions about how you want to live your life. A vast number of food-related illnesses could hinder the quality of your life now, but more likely, into the future. However, it is not only about the unhealthy foods you eat but also the healthy foods you do not eat. According to an article in the Centers for Disease Control and Prevention (CDC) (n.d.), only 10% of adults consume sufficient amounts of fruits and vegetables. With men in general, young adults and low-income earners make up most of the 90%.

List of Micronutrients That People Are Commonly Malnourished In

Fruits, vegetables, and other whole foods contain larger volumes of macronutrients, vitamins, and minerals required to maintain optimum health and bodily functioning. Unfortunately, whenever you choose to grab a pack of candy, you do not get to think about fruits. A lot of fruits carry nutritional value and can never be replaced by sugar which tastes like fruit. According to a document published by WIC (2018), there are well over 300 diseases related to malnutrition. However, only about a dozen make up the most common list. Malnutrition can result from lacking macronutrients like protein, as with kwashiorkor. It can also be due to a lack of certain minerals or vitamins like Iodine or Vitamin A. Below are some of the vitamins and minerals that are most common, some of their common sources, as well as how to detect the deficiency.

Calcium

Calcium is a mineral crucial for every cell in the body. However, it is especially good for bone and teeth growth in children and maintenance in adults. Calcium is regulated in the blood, and excess is stored in the bones. Whenever the body lacks calcium, it will take it from the bones. According to writer and nutritionist Adda Bjarnadottir (2019), "calcium serves as a signaling molecule. Without it, your heart, muscles, and nerves would not be able to function." Some signs of calcium deficiency are tingling or numbness of the fingertips, irregular heart rhythms, and osteoporosis (brittle and fragile bones).

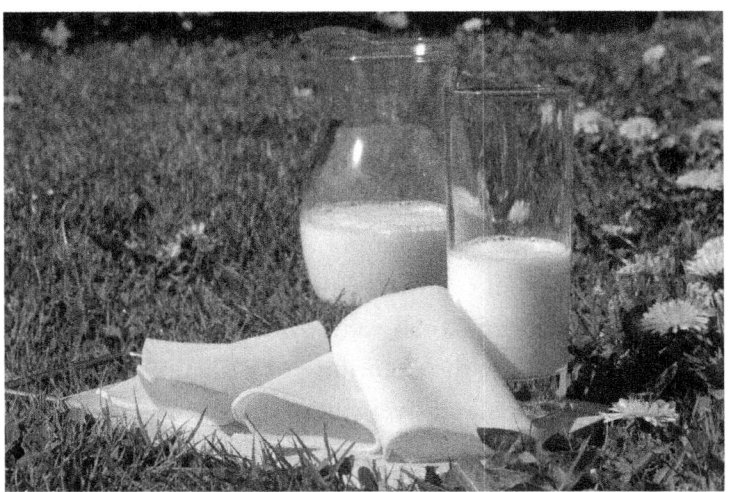

Some of the best sources of calcium include:

- Milk, particularly cow's milk, but almond milk has a significant amount too. Other milk products like yogurt and cheese will also have calcium.
- Dark green vegetables like kale, spinach, broccoli, and bok choy
- Boned fish like sardines, salmon, and shrimp

- Calcium-fortified orange juice is another excellent vegan source of this nutrient.

Folate

Also known as folic acid, this is another type of vitamin B essential for synthesizing RNA and DNA. This is a crucial vitamin for pregnant women and can help prevent congenital disabilities related to the brain and spine. In pregnant women, folate deficiency can cause a decrease in the body's number of cells and enlarged red blood cells, which causes neural tube defects in developing fetuses. In children, folate deficiency can result in poor growth and megaloblastic anemia, which is abnormally large red blood cells. Generally, symptoms of low folate include irritability and fatigue, diarrhea, and tongue tenderness.

You can receive folate from:

- Beans, peanuts, and sunflower seeds
- Whole grains like brown rice, oatmeal, popcorn, as well as whole-wheat bread and pasta
- Dark green leafy vegetables like spinach, kale, and Swiss chard
- Some proteins like eggs and liver (if you are pregnant, avoid the latter)

Iodine

Iodine is essential for your thyroid functioning, which is responsible for growth, brain development, and bone strength. The thyroid is also involved in regulating the metabolic rate, protein synthesis, and enzyme activity. In children, iodine deficiency is especially concerning as it can result in poor growth and even mental retardation. In adults, one of the most familiar symptoms is an enlarged thyroid gland, referred to as a goiter. But patients may also experience breathing difficulties, an irregular increase in heart rate, and weight gain. In some countries, salt is required by law to include iodine, which has resulted in decreased deficiencies.

Some excellent sources of iodine include:

Seaweed such as kelp, kombu, and nori. However, I do not think this is number one on anyone's grocery list, so the next best thing is:

- Fish and shellfish like cod, shrimp, canned tuna, and oysters
- Dairy products like milk, cheese, and yogurt
- Some meat and animal products like chicken, beef liver, and eggs

Iron

Iron is a mineral that is key to the functioning of red blood cells and the transportation of oxygen from the lungs to other organs. There are two types of iron. The first is heme iron which is found in animal products, especially red meat, and is easily absorbed into the body. The second, non-heme iron, is located in animal and plant products but is difficult to absorb. Iron deficiency is highly prevalent, affecting over 25% of people globally (Bjarnadottir, 2019). But the people at more risk are women who are menstruating or pregnant, children, and those following a vegan or vegetarian diet (as they only get non-heme iron which the body cannot easily absorb). Therefore, vegans and vegetarians could benefit significantly from increasing vitamin C in their diets, which helps with iron absorption.

The most common illness that arises due to iron deficiency is anemia. This is because the body does not make enough red blood cells, so not enough oxygen gets transported through the body. Symptoms usually include:

- Fatigue
- Headaches

- A weak immune system
- Difficulty breathing
- Pale skin
- Cold hands and feet
- Swollen tongue
- Brittle nails or nails that are spoon-shaped
- Impaired cognitive functioning

Some people have even reported weird cravings for things like dirt.

Iron can be found in:

- Red meat (beef, lamb, and pork) and organ meat such as livers
- Shellfish such as clams, oysters, and mussels
- Pumpkin, sesame, and squash seeds
- Dark green vegetables like broccoli, kale, and spinach

Magnesium

Magnesium is a critical component in over 300 enzyme reactions, making it essential for protein synthesis, muscle and nerve function, blood sugar regulation, blood pressure regulation, as well as bone and teeth health. A present disease like type 2 diabetes, osteoporosis, heart disease, or drug addiction may make magnesium absorption difficult, leading to deficiency. Deficiencies in healthy individuals are less common but not completely unheard of overall. Low magnesium can cause a lack of energy, loss of appetite, nausea, and vomiting. In more severe patients, numbness, tingling, muscle cramps, seizures, abnormal heart rhythms, and personality changes have been reported.

Some of the best sources of magnesium include:

- Whole grains like oats, whole-wheat bread, and buckwheat

- Nuts like almonds, cashews, and Brazil nuts
- Dark chocolate
- Dark leafy vegetables, which should not come as a surprise

Potassium

This is another mineral essential for the functioning of multiple bodily systems, including the heart, nerves, and muscles. Potassium is key to transporting nutrients into various cells while removing waste. It has the opposite effect as salt when it comes to blood pressure. Essentially it assists in regulating blood pressure, ensuring it does not get too high or stay high for too long. One could lose significant amounts of potassium for a short period if you are experiencing vomiting, diarrhea, or excessive sweating. Potassium levels could also decrease if you are consuming antibiotics, laxatives, diuretics, or excessive amounts of alcohol. However, some severe causes of potassium deficiency are chronic illnesses like kidney disease. Some low potassium symptoms include tingling and numbness, muscle weakness, twitching or cramps, constipation, and heart palpitations.

Potassium can be found in several great-tasting foods, such as:

- Bananas are one of the most versatile fruits ever.
- All types of milk should have potassium, but coconut milk has the most, and almond milk has the least.
- Legumes such as kidney beans, lentils, and peas

Zinc

The body only needs small amounts of zinc to function. However, it is involved in creating DNA, cell metabolism, healing damaged tissue, and supporting overall immune system health. Zinc is found in almost all food groups, so if you are deficient in it, you have to miss out on many decent meals (even processed ones). Nevertheless, deficiency is still possible, and symptoms include a weakened immune system, hair loss, slow wound healing, eye, and skin lesions, as well as stunted growth in children. As mentioned, zinc can be found almost everywhere, including:

- Whole grains
- Dairy products
- Meat
- Legumes
- Nuts
- Some fruits and vegetables (Although these contain relatively small amounts, then again, that is all your body needs.)

Vitamin A

This is a fat-soluble vitamin that is necessary for vision. It also promotes healthy skin, bones, teeth, and cell membranes. There are two forms of vitamin A. The first is preformed vitamin A which can be found in animal products like meat, fish, poultry, and dairy. The second is pro-vitamin A, such as beta carotene, found in fruits and vegetables. Vitamin A deficiency can cause temporary and permanent eye damage, including blindness. It also suppresses "immune function and increases mortality, especially among children and pregnant or breastfeeding women" (Bjarnadottir, 2019). Most people who follow a Western diet are not at high risk of vitamin A deficiency. It is primarily a problem in developing countries. Still, some cases do occur even in first-world countries.

Vitamin A can be found in:

- Organ meat such as beef liver
- Fish liver oil
- Sweet potatoes

- Carrots (the rumors are true; carrots help you see better)
- Dark green, leafy vegetable, making an appearance once again

Vitamin B6

Vitamin B6 is involved in over 100 enzyme reactions and is vital for processing the three macronutrients, fats, carbohydrates, and protein. It is critical for developing the brain and nerves and supports the immune system. Vitamin B6 is also incredible for skin health. A lot of symptoms of deficiency show up in the skin first, like dermatitis (skin inflammation), a red, scaly skin rash, and cracks on the side of the mouth. Some patients may experience microcytic anemia (when the red blood cells are smaller than usual and not receiving enough oxygen), a swollen tongue, depression, and confusion. Some excellent sources of vitamin B6 are chicken, tuna, potatoes, and bananas.

Vitamin B12

Vitamin B12 is involved in producing red blood cells, DNA synthesis, and neurotransmitter (such as dopamine) function. Also referred to as cobalamin, this is a water-soluble vitamin that every cell in the body needs in order to function. The people at higher risk of developing vitamin B12 deficiency are vegans and vegetarians, as this nutrient can only be sufficiently found in meat products. People who have received weight loss surgery are also at risk as "the procedure makes it difficult for the body to extract the nutrient from the food" (Bowers & Lawler, 2021, para. 6). Finally, the elderly are also at risk as the ability of the body to absorb this nutrient gets worse with age.

Something else that makes the absorption of vitamin B12 more complicated is that it requires the help of a protein called intrinsic factor. If someone lacks this protein, they will need vitamin B12 injections or have to take higher doses of supplements containing this nutrient. This also has to be monitored as excessive amounts of the vitamin can harm the body. Nevertheless, in severe cases, vitamin B12 deficiency will cause megaloblastic anemia, fatigue, numb hands, legs, or feet, constipation, weight loss, difficulty walking and balancing (due to the malfunctioning of dopamine), swollen tongue, memory loss, and difficulty thinking.

Vitamin B12 can be found in:

- Shellfish such as oysters and clams
- Animal products (meat, organ meat, dairy, and eggs)
- Plant-based milk and supplements are the next best alternatives.

Vitamin C

Commonly known for its protection against colds and flu, vitamin C can do much more. It also forms blood vessels, ligaments, skin, muscle, and collagen in bones. It is necessary to grow and repair tissues within the body and heal wounds and form scar tissue on the outside. Vitamin C reduces one's risk of high blood pressure, heart disease, and other chronic diseases. The most significant sign of vitamin C deficiency is scurvy which causes patients to be extremely tired, inflamed and bleeding gums, severe joint pain, and weakened connective tissue within the body. Vitamin C is found in:

- Citrus fruits like oranges, mandarin, and lemons
- Fruits like strawberries, blackcurrants, and kiwi
- Vegetables like broccoli, brussels sprouts, and potatoes

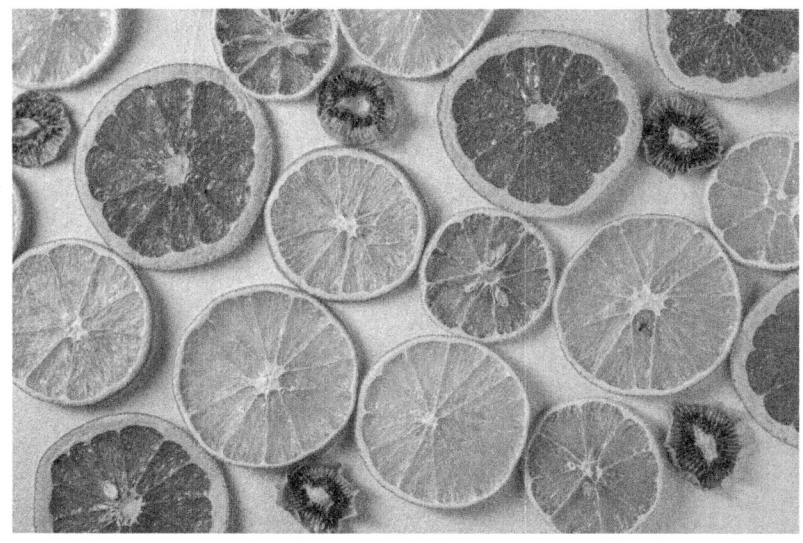

Vitamin D

Vitamin D is a fat-soluble nutrient that tells cells in the body what to do: notably, they turn genes on and off. It is also good for immune functioning, cell growth, and the reduction of inflammation and is believed to prevent some cancers. Vitamin D is key to bone health, and deficiency can lead to bone softening (osteomalacia) and bone pain. Some patients have also reported fatigue, muscle pain, and mood swings. In children, vitamin D deficiency is likely to lead to rickets, characterized by poor growth and soft bones. Exposure to sunlight is the best source of this essential nutrient, and diet alone will never be sufficient to support the recommended amounts.

Nevertheless, vitamin D can be found in:

- Red meat and liver
- Oily fish like salmon, mackerel, and sardines
- Egg yolks (Well, it is a good thing these are natural flavor enhancers.)

List of Diseases Caused by Consuming Unhealthy Foods

Too much sodium, sugar, and unhealthy fats can adversely affect the body over time. You may not see it now, but as the body ages, we are unable to fight off diseases easily, and the compound effect of highly processed foods starts to take its toll. According to an article posted in *U.S. Right To Know* (n.d.), "the government estimates that about half of all American adults—117 million people—have one or more preventable, chronic diseases, many of which are related to poor quality eating patterns and physical inactivity." It all boils down to the choice I have been alluding to in previous chapters, you can choose to eat healthily and prevent many illnesses. Alternatively, you can continue eating foods that are not good for you and suffer the consequences. Many food-related diseases are easily avoidable, such as obesity, type 2 diabetes, cardiovascular, liver, and kidney diseases, Alzheimer's disease, and even some cancers.

Obesity

Obesity is a disease involving excessive body fat. This puts the patient at risk of getting other diseases and health problems such as diabetes, heart disease, and some cancers. A person is considered obese if they have a BMI of 30.0 or higher. Several factors contribute to the prevalence of the disease, such as genetics, the individual's lifestyle, and their environment. Very few cases of obesity are entirely out of the hands of the individual, for instance, having a pre-existing condition that makes it difficult to lose weight. Most people become obese by eating many unhealthy foods and not getting enough physical activity.

Ultimately, this disease occurs when you take in more calories than you burn daily; the body stores the extra calories as fat. Over time, the fat continues accumulating, not only in your fat cells but around vital organs, limiting their functioning and causing more illness. Some of the factors that contribute to obesity include:

- You are eating a diet with more processed foods and takeaways rather than whole foods (fruits, vegetables, and whole grains, which you cook yourself).

- You are consuming large amounts of liquid calories. For instance, sodas are filled with sugar but do not make you feel full, so you drink more than your body can handle.

- Not getting enough exercise because you commute to work with a vehicle, or even worse now, work from home, so you hardly get off the couch.

- A genetic makeup that makes it easy to gain weight or challenging to lose weight. Your genes affect the amount of fat your body stores, how that fat is distributed, your appetite levels, and how you lose calories during exercise.

- Taking medications such as antidepressants, antipsychotic medicines, diabetes medication, anti-seizure medication, and steroids will lead to weight gain if the patients are not getting enough exercise or eating healthily.

- Sleep troubles like amnesia or getting too much sleep can lead to hormonal changes that make you hungrier more often. You can crave processed foods that will make you feel good.

- Stress, whether at home or work, can make people seek out highly palatable food to make themselves feel better and relaxed. Chronic stress can lead to overeating consistently, which ultimately leads to obesity.

- After quitting smoking, some people try to replace cigarettes with food as a way to calm their feelings of anxiety and sometimes just to keep their hands busy.

Obesity increases one's chances of getting other diseases; strokes, digestive problems, sleep apnea, and osteoarthritis are a few not mentioned previously. It also affects the person's overall quality of life, making them feel depressed, guilty and shameful, and unable to move their bodies effectively should it be severe. People who suffer from obesity are also less likely to achieve career-related goals and more likely to distance themselves from social interactions, leading to loneliness.

Type 2 Diabetes

This is an incurable (yet preventable) disease in which the body is unable to regulate its blood sugar levels and cannot effectively use sugar (also known as glucose) for energy. This means too much sugar flows through the blood, damaging the nervous, immune, and circulatory systems. Symptoms of diabetes occur slowly, and some people can live with the disease without knowing about it for up to two years. If you are concerned that you (or someone you love) may have diabetes; you can look out for the following signs:

- Increased thirst and hunger
- Losing weight without exercising or dieting
- Frequent infections and sores over the body that do not heal quickly
- Frequent urination
- Blurred vision
- Unexplained fatigue
- Numbness or tingling of the hands and feet
- Darkened skin, especially around the neck and armpits

Type 2 diabetes arises from two core problems. First, muscle, fat, and liver cells become resistant to insulin, the hormone released by the pancreas that allows sugar to enter into cells, providing them with energy. With these cells lacking energy, they cannot perform their bodily functions effectively. Second, the sugar that does not get absorbed into the cells travels around the bloodstream, triggering more insulin release. Eventually, the body cannot produce enough insulin to keep up with the amount of sugar in the blood. The excess sugar corrodes the body leading to heart and blood vessel disease; nerve damage in the limbs, heart, and penis; sleep apnea (mainly if the person is also obese); sight and hearing impairments; as well as dementia in older patients.

Being obese puts you at a greater risk of getting type 2 diabetes. Other risk factors to look out for include:

- **Family history**. If you have a parent or sibling with type 2 diabetes, this increases your risk.

- **Race or ethnicity**. Although it is unclear why people of color, including Black people, Hispanic, Native Americans, and Asian people, are more likely to get type 2 diabetes.

- **Pregnancy**. If you developed gestational diabetes when you were pregnant or gave birth to a baby weighing above nine pounds, you are at risk of developing type 2 diabetes.

- **Fat distribution**. You are at greater risk if you typically store fat around your abdomen rather than your hips and thighs.

- **Blood lipid level**s. Low levels of high-density lipoprotein (HDL) cholesterol are often referred to as good cholesterol and sometimes indicate malnutrition. At the same time, high triglycerides (fat lipids) are another risk factor.

Ivan Loses His Leg

Ivan had been living with type 2 diabetes for over five years when he received the shocking news that the doctors did not think there was much else they could do for his leg and would have to amputate it. Initially, he was angry. He felt that as a man of color, they were probably discriminating against him, trying to break another Black man down. If that was the goal, they had certainly achieved that, Ivan thought, breathing heavily. He began reflecting on the past few months, trying to think back on what went wrong, but could not pin it on anything or anyone. He remembered how much pain he had been in, and a weird sense of relief came to him as he imagined the pain would no longer be a part of his life.

After several minutes, his chest closed up, his palms began to sweat, and he was overcome with this overwhelming feeling of fear and failure. He understood that he would lose his job at the factory. The payout, he imagined, would only be enough to cover a few months' rent. After that, he would be completely broken. He imagined how disappointed his wife would be in him. She told him several times to get his leg checked out, but he never listened. The "I told you so" look on her face was going to be unbearable. The look of disappointment on the faces of his three young children when their father can no longer provide them with their basic needs will be his end.

They would be here to visit him any second. He considered sending a message saying they should not come to the hospital and needed some time to process everything, but that would just make them panic more, and he did not want that. Instead, he kept rehearsing his apology statement, imagining how his wife would react to each account, then refining it to better reflect how sorry he was. He hated that he would be a burden to the people he was meant to protect from illness and financial troubles, yet he would be bringing them both as soon as he left this bed.

When his family arrived, he tried to put on a brave face. The oldest of his three kids started crying immediately; she knew just how much life was about to change. The younger two did not fully understand, but they could read the room was filled with fear and panic, and they were tense, unlike their usual selves. "I am sorry," Ivan whispered to his wife. She told him that they would be okay. Ivan tried to explain himself, but she told him to save his strength because they would be okay. Ivan knew she was just trying to be strong for him and the kids, but he kept quiet; this would give him more time to practice his apology.

Cirrhosis

Every time the liver gets damaged, it tries to heal itself, and during this process, scar tissue forms. Cirrhosis is a late stage of scarring of the liver, which eventually makes it difficult for the liver to perform its functions. Unfortunately, cirrhosis is usually not diagnosed until the late stages, at which point it is irreversible and potentially life-threatening. Some symptoms individuals can look out for include fatigue; loss of appetite; nausea; weight loss; confusion and slurred speech; swelling of the legs, ankles, and feet; itchy skin or redness of the palms; yellow discoloration of the skin and eyes; spider-like blood vessels visible on the skin; and fluid build up in the abdomen.

Various factors contribute to cirrhosis related to pre-existing conditions and lifestyle choices. For instance, alcohol abuse, consuming a high-fat diet, and risky behavior such as sharing needles or having unprotected sex could increase your chances of contracting hepatitis B and C. If you are obese and diabetic, this can also increase your chances of getting cirrhosis. As mentioned, cirrhosis is potentially life-threatening, and it can lead to several other complications like:

- **Hepatic encephalopathy.** This refers to the accumulation of toxins in the brain. As the liver cannot clear toxins in the blood, these can circulate through the body and form in the brain leading to mental confusion, concentration issues, and eventually unresponsiveness or a coma.

- **Liver cancer.** Cirrhosis can also increase the chances of the patient getting liver cancer.

- **Acute-on-chronic cirrhosis**. This is multi-organ failure due to cirrhosis. However, it is still unclear how this comes about.

- **Bleeding.** This involves multiple layers. First, cirrhosis leads to high blood pressure in the veins that supply blood to the liver. Then, blood is redirected to smaller veins, but these cannot handle the pressure and burst, which leads to severe bleeding. Next, due to its existing damage, the liver cannot create enough clotting factors, so the bleeding does not stop. Finally, high blood pressure may also form in the esophagus and stomach, and the patient risks severe internal bleeding and death.

Chronic Kidney Disease

Also known as chronic kidney failure, this involves the loss of kidney function over time. The kidney's primary function is to remove waste and excess fluids from the blood through the urine. With chronic kidney disease, these fluids, wastes, and electrolytes accumulate in the blood and body. If detected early enough, treatment can sometimes be effective by managing the cause. There are several causes of chronic kidney disease. Like previous diseases mentioned, these can be pre-existing conditions or related to how you have been living your life. Some of the illnesses discussed previously, like diabetes, obesity, and heart disease can lead to kidney failure. Smoking and high blood pressure (often caused by stress) are lifestyle choices that also play a role.

Chronic kidney disease might only present symptoms at the later stages of its development. At this time, some of the signs you can look out for are:

- Nausea and vomiting
- A loss of appetite and overall weakness
- Troubles sleeping or staying focused when awake
- Urinating less or more than usual
- Swelling of the feet and ankles
- Dry, itchy skin
- Muscle cramps
- Uncontrollable high blood pressure
- Shortness of breath due to fluid accumulation in the lungs
- Chest pain due to fluid accumulation in the heart

Heart Disease

Also known as cardiovascular disease, heart disease refers to a broad range of illnesses that affect the heart. Most heart diseases can be prevented and treated by living a healthy lifestyle and avoiding smoking, processed foods, stress, and inactivity. The exact cause and the subsequent symptoms of each heart disease will vary, but if detected early, treatment is possible. Fortunately, symptoms are often undeniable, and should you have heart disease; there are often vivid signs:

- **Coronary artery disease**. This is a type of heart disease affecting the blood vessels. Fat builds up in the arteries leading to chest pain, tightness, or overall discomfort in the chest; shortness of breath, pain in the neck, jaw, upper abdomen, or back; as well as numbness, weakness, or pain in the limbs due to narrowed blood vessels.

- **Heart arrhythmias**. This is when the heart beats at irregular intervals, too slow, or too fast. This could signify another heart disease like coronary artery disease or valvular heart disease. It could also be due to diabetes, stress, high blood pressure, smoking, drug and alcohol abuse, and some over-the-counter medications, dietary supplements, and herbal remedies. Besides the beating of the heart itself, other symptoms to look out for include fluttering in the chest or pain, shortness of breath, dizziness, or fainting (even if it is lightheadedness).

- **Congenital heart defects**. This is one of the heart diseases you can be born with and is not caused by lifestyle choices. Severe defects are spotted soon after birth and can include pale gray or blue skin color, swelling in the legs, abdomen, or around the eyes, and shortness of breath during feedings. Less severe cases are noticed later in childhood and adulthood through swelling of hands, feet, and ankles, shortness of breath, or being tired too quickly during exercise and physical activity.

- **Cardiomyopathy**. This refers to the enlarging of the heart muscle caused by genetics, other heart diseases, an abnormal buildup of proteins, and in rare cases—an unknown reason. Symptoms include shortness of breath with physical activity but even when resting; irregular and rapid heartbeats; dizziness, lightheadedness, or fainting; as well as swelling of the legs, ankles, and feet. Early-stage symptoms are often unavailable, so cardiomyopathy is usually detected when the condition is terrible.

- **Endocarditis**. This type of heart infection is caused by bacteria, viruses, or parasites affecting the inner lining of the heart chambers. Symptoms include fever, fatigue, dry or persistent cough, shortness of breath, irregular heartbeat, swelling in the legs or abdomen, and unexplained skin rashes or spots.

- **Valvular heart disease**. This is caused by damage to the heart valves due to birth defects, heart infections, or connective tissue disorders. Once damaged, the valves can narrow, start leaking or be unable to close effectively. Symptoms depend on which of the four valves is not working and can include chest pain, irregular heartbeat, shortness of breath, fatigue, fainting, and swollen feet or ankles.

Tyler Has a Stroke

Tyler was only 43 when he had a stroke. He knew he was at risk. He felt considerably old, did not eat healthily, had a highly stressful office job, and exercise was like a foreign topic. However, he did not think it was going to happen to him. His parents died in a tragic car accident over a decade ago, so no one he knew had suffered from heart disease before. You always hear stories about people suffering from a stroke or heart attack. All those things seem like things that happened on television or to others, not you or anyone close to you. As it happened, Tyler was not sure what was happening, it felt like he was just extremely tired, too tired to move his left leg forward, so the next sensible move was to drop to the floor.

When he awoke at the hospital, could finally make sense of the world, and received his diagnosis, he remained silent for a long time. He had not even tried to talk but just intrinsically knew that his speech would likely be impaired. When the nurse came to check in on him to run a few assessments, she probed him to talk, which confirmed his initial assumption. Tyler could not even remember simple words that had been part of his vocabulary over the past four decades. This was now starting to concern him, and his easy-going temperament was being replaced by one of panic. He was constantly seeking the following answer but could not always get it. The medical team assigned to work with him tried to reassure him that everything would be okay. However, he felt it was only their job to provide such assurance when the reality of his situation was very different.

Physical therapy to restore his health was a long, painful and expensive excursion. His speech was the first to improve, probably because he had always been good with words. The left side of his neck and shoulder gained movement but always felt stiff if he would even go a few minutes without moving it. So, he would set 15-minute reminders to shift his neck and shoulders just so those muscles could remember that they were still needed. His left leg gained feeling but not full mobility. Even after months of physical therapy, he had a limp and a bit of pain in his leg muscles. Although he described the pain as coming from deep within the muscles, he could not exactly pinpoint where.

As an only child and unmarried man, Tyler longed for support during these trying times. He had a few friends and colleagues who showed him a lot of support, but they had to leave and attend to their own families. If he could get a do-over, he imagined he would marry the last woman he had fallen in love with about seven years back. They would have kids running around by now, giving him a reason to live. He would have home-cooked meals on most days and a support system to bring him hope in the face of the hopeless. Tyler imagined his suffering would be eased if only he made a few minor changes back in the day. However, this is today, and there seemed to be very little that he could do.

Alzheimer's Disease

Alzheimer's is an incurable neurological disorder resulting in the shrinking of the brain and causing brain cells to die. Once detected, treatment can be provided to slow down the progression of the disease. However, eventually, the patient will develop memory impairment, lose their ability to function, and eventually lead the brain to experience dehydration, malnutrition, or infection, resulting in death. The exact causes are not clearly understood, but scientists know that it has to do with proteins in the brain becoming toxic, impairing the regular functioning of the neural system. Significant evidence points to lifestyle choices such as diet and physical activity (or rather the lack thereof), which causes individuals, especially as they grow older, to develop Alzheimer's.

The malfunctioning of the brain leads to:

- **Memory loss**. This is the key sign of Alzheimer's disease, in which the person forgets recent events and conversations. Eventually, they will repeat questions or comments, misplace possessions and leave them in irrational places, forget familiar places and people or the names of family members, and have difficulty identifying everyday objects or finding the right words to express themselves.

- **Flawed reasoning**. People with Alzheimer's tend to find concentrating and multitasking difficult. Reasoning and thinking, especially regarding intangible concepts like numbers, become challenging. So, managing their finances, paying bills, and even recognizing numbers becomes impossible.

- **Irrational decision-making**. Making decisions and judgments even in everyday circumstances becomes a problem.

Social interactions become awkward, and they would struggle to react to traffic or onions burning on the stove.

- **An inability to remember sequences**. Patients lose the ability to plan and perform routine tasks, especially ones involving recognizing particular steps like cooking a meal, getting dressed, or playing a card game.

- **Changes in behavior and personality**. All the changes in the brain can lead the person to experience changes in their typical behavior and temperament. They may develop depression, apathy, and mood swings; social withdrawal, a distrust for people, signs of aggressiveness and irritability toward others; changes in sleeping patterns and getting lost while wandering; delusions; and a loss of inhibitions.

Cancer

Cancer is a large group of diseases in which body cells divide uncontrollably and begin to permeate and destroy normal body cells and tissues. A cell becomes cancerous when it changes or mutates the DNA within the cell. The DNA inside a cell contains a group of individual genes, each with instructions that tell the cell what to do, including when to grow and divide. A cancerous cell cannot receive these instructions clearly and can grow and divide at levels the body cannot handle. Cancerous cells can travel to any part of the body, sometimes attacking multiple tissues and organs. Symptoms are often hard to detect and will vary depending on the type of cancer present. According to an article published in Mayo Clinic (2021), some signs include:

- Persistent indigestion or uneasiness after eating
- Changes in bowel movements and bladder habits
- Unintended weight loss or gain

- Extreme tiredness
- Challenges with swallowing foods and beverages
- A sudden husky voice
- Persistent fevers, coughing, sweating at night, and trouble breathing
- Unexplained muscle and joint pain
- A lump that can be felt under the skin
- Changes to the skin like yellowing, darkening, or redness; sores that refuse to heal; and changes to existing bodily moles
- Bleeding and bruising that occur randomly

A large body of evidence from Better Health Channel (2021) and Mayoclinic (2021) articles points to diet and lifestyle choices contributing to and preventing the growth of cancer cells. Foods to avoid include highly processed foods that provide no fiber; heavily salted and pickled foods; red fatty meats and processed meats; and alcohol. If possible, you might also want to avoid supplements and enjoy the nutrients from natural foods instead. On the other hand, leafy green vegetables, carrots, tomatoes, whole grains, citrus fruits, and cruciferous vegetables (broccoli, brussels sprouts, cabbage, etc.) should make it to the top of your next grocery run.

Am I Scaring You?

You are right; I am trying to scare the living fat out of you. It would be best if you were scared. Losing your quality of life or potentially your entire life because you refuse to take care of your body is not something that should be taken lightly. Yet, so many people still do. You do not want to wait until you get your legs amputated or have to poop in a bag attached to your waist before you open your eyes to the dangers of unhealthy eating and not giving your body enough nutrients. Nor do you want to wait until you are confined to your bed or eat out of a feeding tube (unable to enjoy any type of food) before making the necessary changes to your life. Think about the things you could achieve with more mental clarity and energy. If that does not help, think about yourself on your deathbed, regretting your choices, feeling sad because there is still so much you have not done, and you are not even 50.

Bella Fights Against the Odds

Bella was nearing 30. While other people that age were worried that they did not have enough cars and status just yet, she was concerned that her life as she knew it would be over in about five years, give or take. Bella was afraid she would be diagnosed with Rheumatoid Arthritis. Her mom was diagnosed when she was 34, and her oldest brother recently received the news at 36. Although Bella understood that not everyone in the family would get the diagnosis, she feared that she would because her bone enamel (as diagnosed by a doctor) was already weak. Bella accepted her destiny for a while and awaited the dreaded 30s.

One day, she came across a podcast on preventing autoimmune diseases. She was taken by surprise because, from her understanding, autoimmune diseases were neither preventable nor curable. Nevertheless, she listened attentively. The nutritionist on the podcast spoke about how healthy eating and living have been shown to reduce the genetic markers that lead to some autoimmune disorders. Bella found more research and internet content with similar sentiments—if she cared for her health, she might not be a victim. Bella made it her mission to reach 40 without any signs or symptoms of the disease. She started taking care of her body in a more thoughtful manner. She has been eating well, getting rid of sugar from her diet, and even attempting to get her family on board, although they were not necessarily keen.

Bella is only 32 right now, but she is feeling great. Despite her efforts, she still fears that the diagnosis will come, but she does not want to regret not trying. She imagines she would feel better being told she had the disease when she had done everything within her power to prevent it. Rather than if the diagnosis came, and she can only wish she had tried harder. So, for now, enjoying home-cooked meals, eating a lot of green leafy vegetables, and performing low-impact exercises, as much of the research has pointed to, is her best chance at survival, and she would be happy to take those chances.

Key Takeaways

- There are two critical consequences to your unhealthy life. 1). Most unhealthy foods do not contain enough micronutrients, and 2). The high volumes of additives in unhealthy foods lead to autoimmune diseases and other illnesses presented by a weakened immune system.

- Most people do not get the recommended amounts of vitamins and minerals daily because they do not eat enough whole foods containing these micronutrients. The result is malnutrition, and some of the most common ones are deficiencies in one of the following: Vitamins A, B6, B12, C, and D, as well as calcium, folate, iodine, iron, magnesium, potassium, and zinc.

- One of the most common autoimmune diseases that stem from overeating unhealthy foods is obesity. Obesity is the leading risk factor in many other illnesses like type 2 diabetes, heart disease, cirrhosis, chronic kidney disease, Alzheimer's disease, and cancer. However, even if you are not obese or overweight but eat a diet rich in sugar, salt, and fat, these diseases are highly likely to catch up to you.

- This should induce a significant deal of fear in you as these deficiencies and diseases can become severe and lead to an early death. The question you should ask yourself is, what are you willing to do to make healthy eating a more prominent aspect of your life?

CHAPTER 4

RESEARCH STUDIES ON ENJOYING HEALTHY FOOD

For the past couple of years, decades perhaps, you have been conditioned to enjoy unhealthy food and view healthy food as some punishment, something you have to do when you have no other option. But face it, we are always met with options, with 24-hour convenience stores, packaged goods that mimic the real thing, and "3 for 2" deals that encourage us to stock up. Again, a choice is always available, so you can shrug your shoulders and say this is the card you have been dealt. Alternatively, you can take a stand and become more curious about what you put in your pantry and your mouth. The truth is, years of psychological food conditioning will not be undone with a few hours of reading. Although this is a great read, there is admittedly a lot of work to be done beyond just reading and acknowledging the problem.

Nutritionists, health scientists, and big food corporations (for more profitable reasons, of course) have recognized there is a problem and have tried (and continue to try) some new psychological probing to help push us toward a healthier way of living. Their efforts are not always received well, and there are some kinks to the system, but it is potentially a way forward. Some of our deeply rooted attraction toward highly palatable foods can be minimized and eventually ostracized through bias reversal, mental labeling, and memory rehearsal. This is a long-term vision and will take some time for everyone to get on board with it, but it is not impossible.

Bias Reversal

The consequences revealed in the previous chapter are not exactly hot news. Most of that information is freely available, and most people already know some of it to be true. Yet, despite the warnings, we are drawn toward those very food choices that could leave us physically and emotionally scarred—literally in some instances. One of the reasons for this is the perception that unhealthy means tasty, and consequently, healthy equals less tasty, even before we put the goods in our mouths. In a world where pleasure is the ultimate goal, what is perceived as delicious will always win. Raghunathan et al. (2006) ran four experiments and discovered that when analyzing various food items on a spectrum of healthy to unhealthy, "the less the item is portrayed to be, 1) the better is its inferred taste, 2) the more it is enjoyed during actual consumption, and 3) the greater is the preference for it in choice tasks when a hedonic goal is more salient."

This is to say that although people understand that the item is unhealthy, they have this instant belief that it has to be good on the tongue too, and upon consumption, reinforce this belief. Bias reversal is about reversing the idea that unhealthy means tasty, and healthy means bland. Taking into account cultural differences between Americans and the French, this is possible. In a study conducted by Werle et al. (2013), they found that Americans have established a culture with the mindset that unhealthy food implies scrumptiousness. In contrast, people in France have the exact opposite bias. For the French, healthy foods are considered tasty, and unhealthy food is thought of as lacking the right volume of flavor. This is good news because if something such as the meaning of taste is not a universal human quality, this means it comes down to psychology and what we have been taught through the media, with those persistent advertisements.

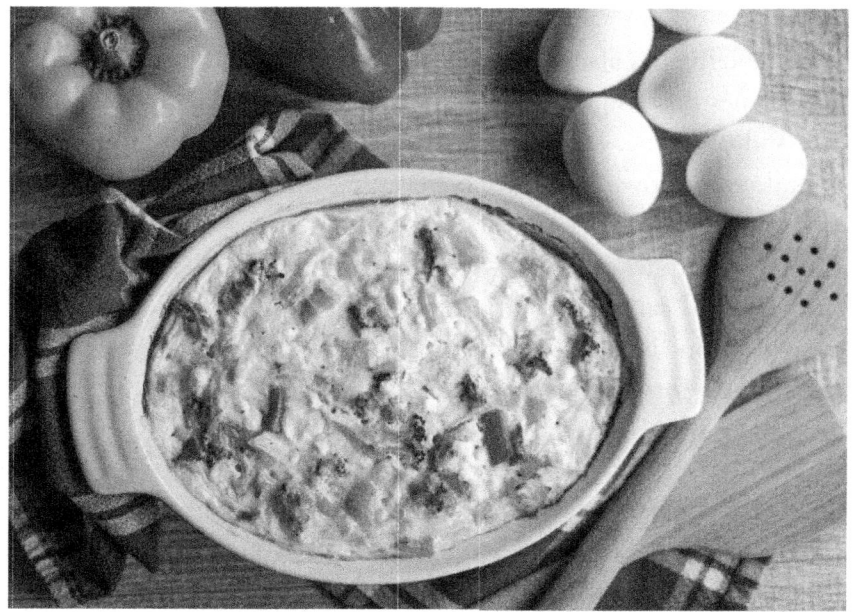

Bias Reversal in Action

Bias reversal will require the cultural influence (through media) that healthy food tastes great. There is no denying that we take to heart whatever we see on television and now on social media apps. Just as big money was being thrown toward making people (particularly in the U.S.) believe that unhealthy food is yummy, often ignoring the consequences, there has to be money spent on making people see the delicious side of fruits, vegetables, and whole grains. Currently, eating healthy is a niche culture, perceived to be only for the wealthy, fitness obsessed, and those trying to save the planet and the animals. It will also require the influence of product labeling and memory rehearsal, two elements that have affected the bias toward the unhealthy in the first place.

Mental Labeling

Food labeling has always been a big part of the food industry; whatever comes on the packaging significantly affects how much people buy and consume. For a highly intelligent species, we are incredibly gullible to our own kind. We believe that other humans will always have our best interests at heart and will never feed us poison simply to feed their pockets. Boy, were we wrong! Even when the "health rush" started, and people became slightly more conscious about what they put in their bodies, those big food companies were leaps ahead of us, forming food labels that further played with our minds, keeping us dumb and fat.

- **The Low-Fat Label**. Fat, in general, has been demonized as the cause of all weight gain issues and other health-related problems. As mentioned, this is only partially true, as healthy fats are necessary for the body's sustenance. The problem with this label is that big food companies used this to trick us into believing the foods were now healthy because they did not have as much fat. However, they added more sugar to the goods to compensate for the loss in fat and flavor. This label also made people think that because there is not as much fat, they would not gain weight if they overeat. It would be like overeating tomatoes, no harm, no foul. We later realized this is certainly not the case. Yet, there is no doubt that the big food companies knew that but did not see the need to inform the consumer as they were now buying more low-fat food options.

- **The Reduced Sodium Label**. Salt has been positively linked to high blood pressure and several other health issues, so health-conscious people decided to reduce their consumption of the mineral. Big food corporations saw the opportunity, created low sodium food options to fill the gap (thank you, finally!), and blasted the good news all over their labels. However, this created the impression that there was not enough salt in the products themselves, and consumers felt the need to add some salt of their own to these products, defeating the whole purpose. Not to put the naivety of the consumer solely on the big food companies, but they should have a moral obligation to explain their labels more clearly. This is something they would never bother to do. They have always had this out-of-sight, out-of-mind outlook on consumer behavior.

- **The Organic Label**. In recent years, organic and natural have become buzzwords in the health and wellness world. Big food companies swooped in again to take advantage of the hype, creating organic and natural products. They knew studies showed that "people perceive food products labeled organic as having fewer calories, having a better nutritional profile than non-organic products, and tasting lower in fat and higher in fiber" (Gloria, 2013, para. 6). What they fail to mention on their labels, however, is that the people's perceptions are wrong and that most of their products, although following organic or natural methods of production, do not necessarily mean they are lower in calories, higher in nutrients, and are always free of chemicals. Some organic products can, in fact, be higher in calories, and some natural products can include trace amounts of chemicals.

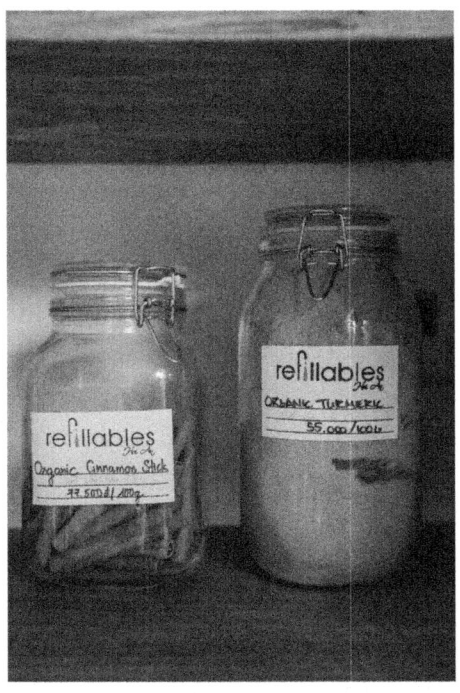

Big food corporations understand the power of the label. However, they have consistently failed the consumer with labeling products adequately and creating products that match the complete perceptions of the consumer. When you read "organic" or "low-fat," you do not want to imagine that it will not mean low calories and low sugar. Those companies feed off your naïve nature, and because it is not like they are hiding anything, they know they can get away with it. Food labeling plays a significant role in our mental perceptions of what we eat, and it could play a massive role in encouraging people to choose healthier food options.

Mental Labeling in Action

Instead of expecting the consumer to do their own research, knowing they will not, food companies should put a greater effort into explicitly labeling their products and detailing all the facts. But that is not the only solution. Because people do not perceive healthy as tasty, knowing that more sugars or calories are packed into a particular product might not make people move away from buying that product, as the food bias is still there. Similarly, knowing something is healthy will not always drive people toward that option because they are concerned with the taste. So, what needs to happen is for the mental labeling of healthy food not to focus on the health aspects of the food but on the taste factors.

In a research study done by Stanford University, the eating behavior of undergraduates in self-dining halls at five different schools was tracked over three months. The menu rotated daily, but each school served the same vegetable dish on the same day of the week, changing only the labels. The label used to explain the vegetable being served would be taste-focused, health-focused, or neutral:

> Taste-focused labels used words that highlighted specific flavors of the ingredients or preparation methods, along with words that suggested a positive experience through excitement, indulgence, tradition, or geographic locations. Health-focused labels communicated the nutritional qualities and health benefits of vegetables. Basic or neutral labels were nondescript. For example, the taste-focused label of "caramelized balsamic and herb vegetable medley" was changed to the health-focused label of "light n' fit vegetables" or just the basic label of "vegetables" (Huber, 2019).

Surprisingly (or maybe not for us anymore), the result was that students were 29% more likely to dish up the taste-labeled vegetables than health-labeled dishes and 14% more likely than the neutral label. So, people would rather have a neutral label than a healthy one. Enforcing the idea of health onto people who are not as concerned with health as they are with hedonics does not help the problems we face with obesity and other food-related illnesses. What will help is playing the mental game, making people see that taste is a big part of even the healthiest foods like vegetables.

You may be wondering if, upon consumption, people will remember that they are still eating vegetables—even if they are "caramelized"—and spit it out. If the results from the above-mentioned study are anything to go by, this should not be the case. The study also revealed that at one of the schools (with no indication as to why they did not observe all the schools on this essential measurement), the students who received the taste-labeled vegetables were 39% more likely to eat the vegetables on their plates in comparison to the health-labeled plates. So, just like people with a bias toward unhealthy foods believe that the unhealthy food tastes great and confirms this belief upon consumption, the same is true when eating healthy foods. Because the label makes you think it should be flavorful, the experience itself will be. It is all a mental game.

Memory Rehearsal

What has been the biggest win for big food corporations? Their ability to make food so memorable that you will come back begging for more. The thing about unhealthy foods is that their enjoyment is so embedded into their fabrication that you remember the foods and get unconsciously pulled toward them. With healthy foods, you need a little more work because, if we were to face it, there is nothing *that* memorable about garlic-glazed green beans. Nevertheless, as mentioned in a study by Robinson et al. (2012), "novel ways to increase liking and intake of food are needed to encourage acceptance of healthier food. How enjoyable we remember food to have been is more likely to be a significant predictor of food choice." Memory rehearsal for healthy foods means actively encouraging the memorable factors about the healthy foods we eat so we can keep those factors in mind next time we are faced with an option. The option to either choose an unhealthy option which we have come to believe will always taste great, or the healthy choice we have now come to enjoy.

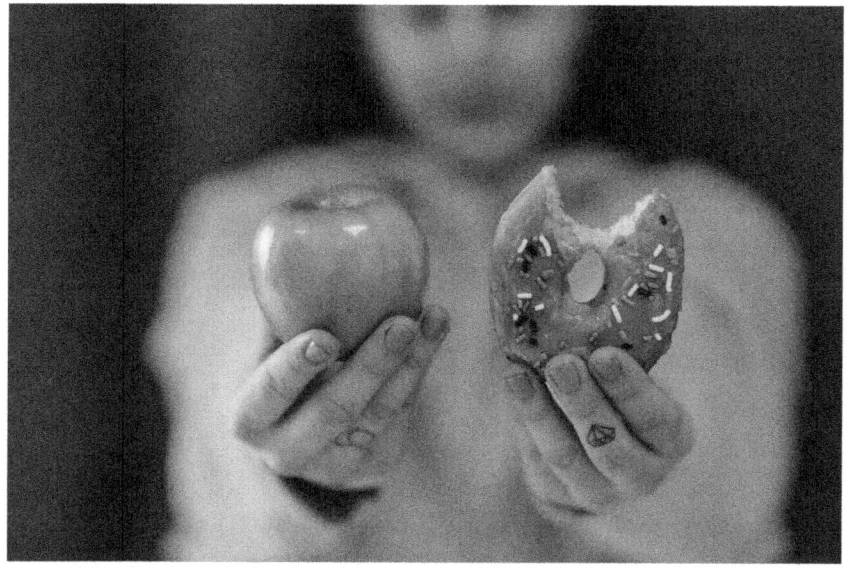

Memory Rehearsal in Action

In the Robinson et al. study, participants were asked to list some elements they enjoyed about a healthy meal immediately after eating it. They discovered that the participants could recall those enjoyable elements long after eating the meal. They also choose to eat those meals (or something similar) when faced with the option to do so later. Without active recall, this is not easily possible. Think about how often you have seen the salad as an alternative to fries as your side option. Yet, you still select fries because you know the hedonic factor of these from years of conditioning. If you want to start having the salad, you cannot simply view it as the healthy alternative you have to eat but rather as the flavorful option you want to eat.

Memory rehearsal has another part to it. You do not only have to do it after eating but as you are eating as well. Pay attention to the salad's different parts: the crispy lettuce, juicy tomatoes, creamy avocado, savory cheese, and cool cucumbers. This helps you remember and enjoy the salad and also enables you to recognize when you are full. One of the things about our eating habits is that we munch away so thoughtlessly that we do not even realize when we are full. Memory rehearsal, mainly as we are eating, can solve another problem we face that contributes to weight gain and obesity. Then, finally, because we remember what we have eaten, we also feel fuller for longer, so we do not have that urge to snack as often. I will touch more on this particular topic later.

Key Takeaways

- Bring about your own bias reversal by actively seeking out media and digital content that shows the benefits and positive aspects of healthy living. You cannot wait for big food companies to pour money into something unless it is benefiting them directly. Plus, the companies currently promoting healthy living are still doing so from a biased view. They exclusively support organic living and plant-based diets, which are more expensive to subscribe to for the average person. So, find your own answers and sources.

- Create your own mental labels for the foods you buy and cook. If you cook some meals in advance and place them in smaller containers, label them as exotically as possible. This will also encourage you and your family to want to eat the leftovers. Mental labeling only goes as far as taste, so do put in a considerable amount of effort to ensure the food tastes good.

- As you eat each meal, implant the food's best qualities into your mind. Pay attention to the dynamic contrast of healthy foods by memorizing the flavors, smell, texture, and any other positive qualities you would want to consider the next time you think of having the same meal or something similar.

- Once you realize you hold the power to change how you perceive your food, you are able to make healthy eating decisions more often. Do not just wait for the food brands to enforce these changes; even if they do, they will not always do so with pure intentions or your best interests at heart.

CHAPTER 5

THE CHALLENGES OF EATING HEALTHY AND ENJOYING HEALTHY FOOD

When the odds are stacked against you, it is hard to find the courage to push beyond what you can see. Being unhealthy, overweight, and physically unfit is not part of anyone's wish list. However, it is part of many people's realities. The urge to become healthy is not likely to be a fad, at least, I hope not. Many people, yourself included, are opening up to what lies behind the counter. No, it is not the last box of Krispy Kreme donuts; it is your dignity. Getting yourself to overcome years of conditioning from a plan that's been set in motion for decades is not meant to be an easy task. The purpose of this book was not to provide you with a simple step-by-step plan for eating well and losing weight. You have already read those books; they do not help much. Not because they are poorly written, but because you were reading them from behind the veil of how food affects you.

With the veil uncovered, you can see highly processed foods for what they really are, not a treat to be enjoyed on your cheat days (of which you still have too many), but rather as goods that should be handled with caution because they could literally cost you your life. There is no denying it; processed foods taste better. I would opt for a slice of carrot cake instead of my carrot sticks any other day. Plus, there is still a lot of work that needs to be done to remove the inherent perception that healthy foods are not delicious and make people believe and see that these can actually be tastier.

Nevertheless, three more issues need to be unraveled, potentially holding you back from being the healthy version of yourself you are striving to be. Some people might not even recognize the barriers to their healthy lifestyle. Again, I am all about uncovering that veil. If you can fully understand what has been standing in your way, you are able to tackle it head-on. It is easy to fight a monster you can see and size up. The three anomalies you must consider fighting are related to the foods themselves, your environment, and your own self-limiting beliefs as they pertain to weight loss and being healthy in general.

Healthy Foods Are More Expensive and Inconvenient to Prepare

Even if we get over the taste hurdle, being healthy and choosing a healthier lifestyle feels more difficult for individuals who lead a busy life or may not have enough money to pay for their basic needs. Let alone consider a healthy meal when there is a more affordable option for themselves and their families. It is another undeniable fact that unhealthy foods do tend to be:

- **Quick.** Preparing a healthy meal for one's family might take several hours. Whereas buying a bucket of wings and fries for everyone to share only takes a few minutes of waiting in the drive-through. Even if you go to a restaurant serving healthy meals, they usually take up to an hour to prepare the food. While you are hungry, try to fill up on water and buttered bread.

- **Accessible.** Finding a fast food joint is not so tricky. In urban areas, there is one at every corner. There are only still a select few places that serve healthy offers. Something else to consider is that not all healthy people are the same and may follow a different diet and nutritional plan. Finding vegan-friendly options is more accessible than keto-friendly or Paleo-friendly options. In contrast, processed foods are friendly to almost everyone.

- **Cheap.** Healthy food options tend to be more expensive, making it difficult for most people to subscribe to that life, even though they may need to. "A comprehensive review of 27 studies in 10 countries found that unhealthy food is about $1.50 cheaper per day than healthy food" (See, 2020, para. 3). For someone who has to feed a large family in a low-income (even middle-income) home, this would not make financial sense.

Making Healthy Eating Affordable and Easier

There are ways to enjoy healthy living that are cost-effective, but they will not necessarily be convenient. The question will now be on you as to whether you need your life to be so convenient that you are willing to risk your health and your family's well-being. In life, there is always going to be a give-and-take situation. You take the easy way out and pay for that with your quality of life. You give a little more effort to being health conscious and enjoy your life well into the future. Keeping this in mind, here are some ways you can be healthy on a budget:

- **Buy frozen fruits and vegetables**. Fresh produce does come with a better taste guarantee, but it only has a shelf life of several days. You will likely end up throwing some of those goods away, wasting money, and spending more. With frozen vegetables, food can stay in the freezer for up to a year while retaining almost all of its nutritional value.

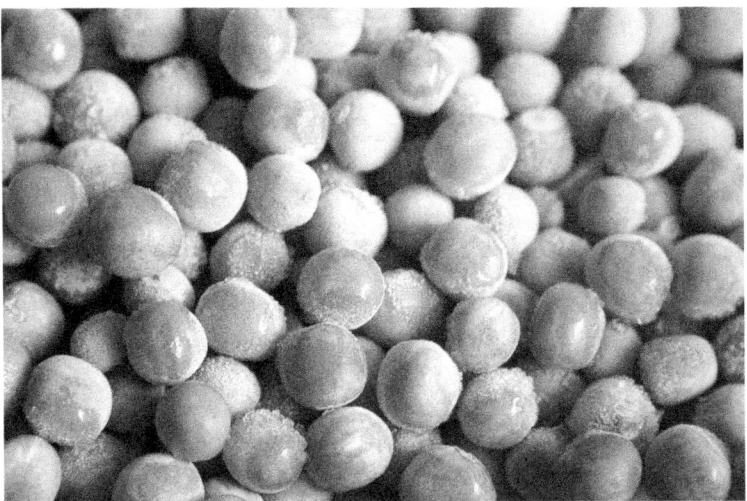

- **Cut up your own fruits and vegetables.** This is not precisely a time-saver, but certainly a money-saver. When you buy pre-cut produce, you get charged for the labor. Sometimes it is best to avoid fruits and vegetables like pineapples and butternuts. Then find alternatives that will be easier to prepare but still contain similar nutrients. You can leave these for special occasions.

- **Do not buy organic.** This is a nice-to-have that does not always live up to the hype and may still include pesticides. They are more expensive than necessary because consumers perceive them to be of much better quality than what they truly are. Instead, choose in-season conventionally farmed fruits and vegetables.

- **Plan your meals for the week.** Buying weekly can help you buy goods required that week alone, even the fresh produce that you know will be necessary and not go to waste. When you plan for the month, you could buy food that is not necessary, and that is how wastage starts. You should also cook your meals in advance and store some in the fridge and freezer. That way, you save time if you are busy and cannot always stand over a stove.

- **Buy your meat in bulk.** This can save you money, and storage in the freezer is easy. For those that do not subscribe to any particular diet, stocking up on protein (natural protein) is good for you and can help you enjoy your healthy lifestyle more.

It Is Not About Changing Your Conditions

It is easy to stand on the sidelines and make excuses. If only you had more time, more money, or lived in an area closer to the farmer's market. You imagine that life will be ten times more manageable if your conditions were to improve. However, often even when conditions improve or change, you still do not. Sasha is an overweight 28-year-old. She is single but has a boyfriend who lives a few hours away, and they plan visits every other weekend. She was a bookkeeper at a small law firm that had to close down during the 2020 pandemic as the leading lawyer passed away (it was a family-owned firm). Sasha was lucky enough to obtain a work from home opportunity a few weeks later.

She was catching up with a friend from her old job, who randomly said the weirdest thing: "You are probably 10 pounds lighter by now," she giggled. "I wish," Sasha responded, "I feel like I have gained 10 pounds instead." After the conversation, Sasha wondered why her friend would say something like that, Sasha's weight had always been a bit of a sensitive subject, and her friend knew that. Then, after a few hours of contemplating the conversations off and on, it hit her. Sasha used to complain about the long commute to and from work. She told her friend several times that was why she did not get a chance to exercise or cook for herself. Plus, the fact that she was not married, she did not even have anyone to cook for, and could not precisely cook three-course meals for herself, she would overeat even more.

Sasha had one of her conditionals changed, but her behavior did not. She was working from home now but still did not exercise or eat healthily. She did not even remember the conditions she had put ahead of her healthy living plans. It is now evident that those were excuses, not obstacles. The sad part is that even after that brutal conversation with her friend, she still did not make any change. Perhaps she was waiting for the marriage proposal before she could start cooking three-course meals. However, it is possible that even if that happens, something else will be standing in her way, similar to how there is always something standing in yours. The truth is, you are your only obstacle. If you want to, you can apply the tips on eating healthy on a budget and get the life you desire.

Healthy Living Is Difficult if Those Around You Are Not Interested

You are the sum of the people you spend the most time with. The people you spend the most time with will ultimately affect the person you become. If those people are unhealthy and have unhealthy behavior, that is bound to rub off on you. Healthy living when you are on your own is tough. When other forces and people are driving you down in the process, this can make things much more complicated. For example, imagine you have to cook for your family, and they refuse to eat the vegetables on their plate because they are used to enjoying fries and nuggets. Suppose you want to go snack-free for a few weeks, but everyone around you is munching on all your favorites; at some point, you are bound to give in to the temptation.

According to an article published in Harvard School of Public Health (2014), "a person's chance of becoming obese increases by 57% if a close friend is obese, 40% if a sibling is obese, and 37% if a spouse is obese… Obesity is contagious."

Bring Your Family and Friends on Board

Bringing this change to your life can be difficult if you are not feeling supported. As the self-help author and motivational speaker Peter Sage always says, your environment will beat your willpower in every situation. He even goes as far as saying that you might have to consider cutting the toxic people out of your life, intentionally holding you back, and finding a circle of friends and supporters who will encourage you to greater heights. This is, of course, easier said than done. Plus, you cannot exactly decide to cut ties with your family simply because they do not want to join your diet. That is selfish on your part too, and a better approach would be to motivate them to see healthy living as the best way to live your lives.

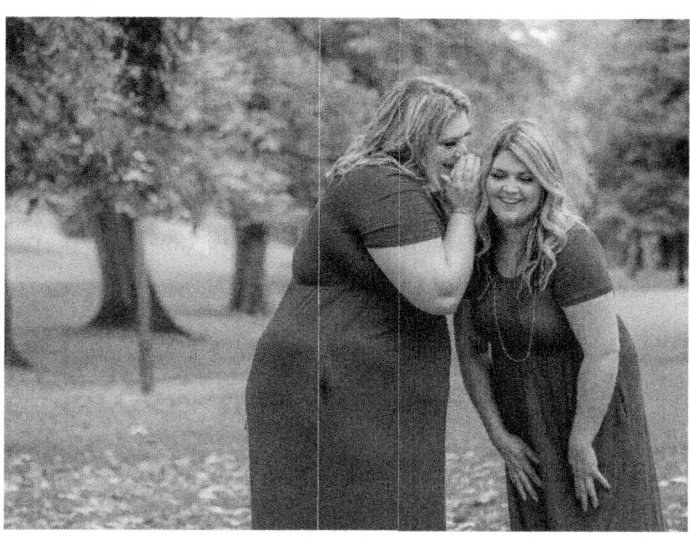

- **Set up a challenge**. This can work great with a friend or spouse. You can create a challenge and hold each other accountable for following through. You are also less likely to cheat on your diet should you know you will have someone to report your missteps to. Set reasonable rewards and punishments for yourselves should you meet or fail to meet your goals.

- **Understand the nutritional needs of others**. You might want everyone around you to be ketogenic or vegan, but just because a diet works for you does not mean it will be best for everyone else. In encouraging those around you to live healthily, encourage them to stay away from processed foods (even the vegan-friendly treats have high levels of sugar at times) instead of trying to convince them that your way of life, in particular, is best.

- **Go outside your immediate circle**. Although it will not be as strong of a support group, having a gym buddy you can talk to about your challenges can keep you grounded for some time. This might be just enough time to curb your unhealthy habits long enough until you are no longer addicted to them.

- **Push yourself with visual cues**. Write down your goals and place them where you and perhaps a few others can see them. Even if they do not join you, they will know that they should not tempt you to go out for ice cream or encourage you to take a break from your exercise when you need to push yourself harder.

How Far Would You Go to Protect the Ones You Love To What Lengths Are You Willing to go to Protect Your Family

Tom married the love of his life while they were still in their 20s. He wanted to provide everything for her, protect her and keep her safe at all costs. His goals were both financial and physical in nature. One morning he woke up in a cold sweat; he had just had the worst nightmare. Two men, bigger and stronger than he was, broke into his home and grabbed his wife. He tried to attack and fight for her, but he was too weak to stop them. Although he was not overweight, he was not physically fit or well-nourished. The criminals took off with the one thing he loved more than anything in this world, and he was left weeping on the floor.

This dream stuck with him long after the nightmare was over. What would happen if someone bigger and stronger than him tried to harm Lisa, he would think to himself over and over again. Those thoughts, fortunately, grew into action. Tom decided he would not let anything like that ruin his life, not when he still had ample opportunity to make the necessary changes. For months, he worked to lose some weight and gain some muscle, challenging himself to work out daily. He had a mantra that if he was not working on his business, he would be working on his body. He avoided all processed foods; ate salted broccoli and boneless chicken breast as his staple.

He received the results he wanted: he was lean and muscular, physically and emotionally ready for anything life wanted to throw at him. Since starting his podcast, *Impact Theory*, Tom has interviewed dozens of health experts and realized there might have been better ways to lose weight and gain muscle than he put himself through. I strongly suggest you listen to some of those interviews; they can be life-changing. However, the moral of this story is that you should find something that motivates you and drives you to take care of your health, as Tom did. It does not have to be a woman or someone other than yourself, but it has to drive you to do the work.

Healthy Living in the Face of Self-Limiting Beliefs

You communicate with yourself at every living moment. Whether consciously or unconsciously, the life you are living right now is the life you have told yourself you should have. It is easy to say you want something, but if your actions and results do not match up, often there is something deeper at play. Self-limiting beliefs can affect any area of your life. You might be very confident in your skills and ability to do your job. This could show up in how you ace job interviews and get headhunted by other organizations. However, when a girl talks to you, you suddenly become as red as a tomato, your glands dry up, and you feel like your chest is about to explode. Not because you cannot handle talking to people, but simply because this specific area of life makes you feel a little awkward, and perhaps you do not feel like you can or should talk to women that way.

You might have a limiting belief system around your weight loss and health journey, making the very thought of finally getting the body you have been dreaming about feel like a hopeless endeavor. Self-limiting beliefs are believed to be rooted in early childhood experiences. They cause you to doubt yourself and your behavior and make you lose faith in the process. The result is that you think you have to switch to another diet or that there is no use trying. The thing about having a self-limiting belief around your appearance is that you could also develop self-limiting beliefs around other areas of your life, making you feel unhappy and potentially lonely.

What You Tell Yourself

What you tell yourself is very important because you wind up believing it. Nevertheless, change does not come from pointing fingers or shrugging your shoulders. You will only be able to make the necessary changes to your lifestyle if you take the time to do so. This means the following self-limiting statements must exit your mind and never make their way back.

- **Being healthy is so hard**. Anything worth having will be hard to achieve. But there is a fine line between being unable to do something and being too lazy to do it. If you have tried losing weight in the past but failed, that happened because you had not been unveiled just yet. Also, it is possible that you gave up on your weight loss goals earlier than you were meant to give up. Sometimes it takes up to 90 days for a new diet to kick in, after which you can start monitoring results. Once you give healthy living a real chance, you will find it is not so hard.

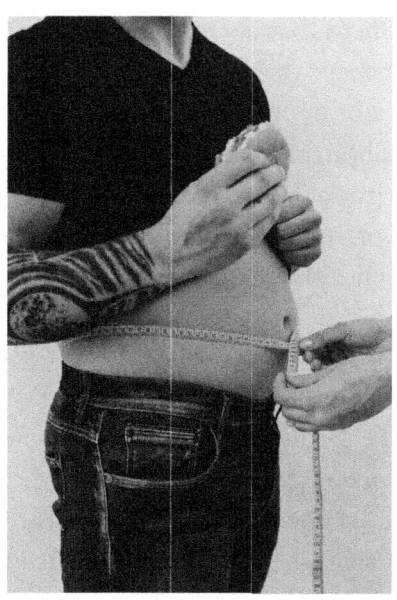

- **This is just how I am.** Perhaps you have always been on the chubby side of life. However, that does not mean that is how you are supposed to be until you die of a heart attack at 40. Unless you have a genetic disorder diagnosed by a professional, you are not allowed to use this excuse. Being born chubby and being fed a lot of fast food as a toddler and young child does not mean you should maintain the status quo. You have a choice as to what goes into your body, and you can decide how you move it.

- **I would rather be fat and happy.** People usually associate the process of weight loss and healthy living with being miserable. Not because skinny people are unhappy, but because the process of going from overweight to average weight is tedious. Plus, if you fail at it (especially a few times), it can start affecting your self-esteem. This leaves you with the belief that you have to remain unhealthy to keep your dignity and the last bit of joy you have left.

- **This is how we are at home.** As mentioned, being part of an environment that encourages unhealthy eating habits can make you believe that is how things are meant to be for you. This could not be further from the truth. You, your parents, and your siblings do not share a hive mind. So, you can break free from their patterns and potentially get them to see that all of you could enjoy more fruitful lives if you each switched to healthy eating.

- **It is inconsiderate not to finish your plate.** Have you ever been told to finish your food because children in Africa are starving? Well, this is one of those quotes that used to get shared to encourage children to finish their plates when they wanted to leave the dining room table early to play. However, you might have taken it on too literally. Plus, your plate now certainly is not as small as the plate you were encouraged to finish when you were a child. You should consider dishing it up on a smaller plate.

What You Do Not Say

Self-limiting beliefs often stem from a place of lack and come with a lot of emotional baggage where the person has been made to believe that they do not deserve to be happy or to seek something that they want. It is not only that you are saying you do not want to or lack the capacity to do it, but rather that you do not think you even deserve to. After years of contemplation, Justin finally decided to seek therapy. He had been chubby as a young body, he lost most of that weight during puberty, but it all came back in his late 20s, going into his early 30s. At the time, there was a lot happening in his life. His mom passed away, and he was overlooked for a promotion for the third time in two years. He had been single for over five years and was not sure what direction to take his life.

The weight gain occurred over several years, like with anyone else. He could tell he was gaining weight, slowly but surely, but it did not always strike him just how bad it actually was. Some people at work and a few of the friends he had left mentioned that he needed to check himself, but they all jokingly brushed it off. Justin was not concerned about his body as much as the mental turmoil he had been going through. He felt himself falling into what he termed a mild depression. He was trying his best to figure out how to get out of that mental slump, sometimes with his face and fingers covered in KFC herbs and spices.

Justin managed to work through some of his problems. He healed from the loss of his mom. He quit his job to work at another company where he had hoped there would be better growth opportunities. He was even considering swiping right on the profile of a few pretty faces. He struggled for a few months to eat healthily and incorporate exercise into his daily lifestyle as this had been something he had not done in years. He decided to get a fitness coach to assist with this. Unintentionally, he found someone who had done sports psychology as part of their training. Their workout sessions were very chatty and felt like a session on the couch, not just in the gym.

"Do you think you deserve to look good?" his coach asked him one afternoon. Justin did not know how to answer and just gave a blank stare. After a few seconds of awkward silence, his coach continued. "Well, you come in here and do some of the work. You talk about your goals and physical aspirations, but something is not adding up."

"I know I have been eating one too many pizzas, but I am doing my best here," Justin felt the need to interject.

"I get it," assured his coach, "and that is exactly what I mean. Your actions and goals are not completely aligned, and it is not because you find this process difficult or anything; otherwise, you would not be coming to these sessions. So it is almost like you do not think you deserve to look good and feel good, so you sabotage your progress and make excuses, and I just want to get to the bottom of it. So, do you think you deserve to look good?"

"Yes?" answered Justin, still unsure what his coach was saying.

"Will you say it as you mean it?"

"Yes."

"I will need a little more than that, Justin."

"Yes, I deserve to look good."

"Then act like it. Whatever you have been telling yourself about this journey you are on, stop it. Focus on those words you have just spoken. Every time you feel the urge to deviate from your goals in any manner, remind yourself that you deserve to look and feel spectacular. There is nothing that will stand in the way of that feeling."

Justin did precisely that, and it was not until weeks after this incident that he realized what the coach had been going on about on that fateful day. Self-limiting thoughts and beliefs creep up on you unexpectedly, challenging your willpower and taunting you into submission. You have to start recognizing them for what they are and override them with a firm belief that you deserve well-being, abundance, and a life of joyfulness.

Key Takeaways

- Unhealthy eating is quick to prepare, accessible almost everywhere, and more affordable. You cannot do much about the inconvenience that comes along with healthy eating, but what you can do is make it more affordable by buying frozen instead of fresh fruits and vegetables, chopping up your own fruits and vegetables, buying in-season instead of organic produce, buying your meat in bulk, and planning and cooking your meals for the week in advance.

- You must ensure your family and friends support your health journey, or they may inadvertently hold you back. Ask your spouse or friend (the person you spend the most time with) to join you on the 10-day detox challenge or similar. Please encourage your family to find the best diet for them, and support each other. Find a gym buddy or accountability partner outside your immediate circle if you need to.

- A vast array of self-limiting beliefs holds you back from being your best healthy version. You may believe that being healthy is difficult, that it is just part of your nature and genetics, or that you can be happy even if you are overweight. The truth is, these beliefs are centered on your self-confidence, and continuing to believe them leaves you less vulnerable than imagining yourself doing something beyond your comfort zone.

- Remember that you deserve to be truly happy and look great. This is only possible when you push past the beliefs you hold for yourself and do not allow your environment and circumstances to hold you back. Tell yourself daily that you deserve to look good; say it until you believe it and embody it with your actions.

CHAPTER 6

PRACTICAL TIPS TO EATING HEALTHIER

Knowing everything you know now, what do you intend to do differently? Remember that knowledge without action goes wasted, and you have come too far (reading this book and in life) to have it all wasted with inaction. I do not expect you to be a health nut tomorrow, but I hope you take steps toward enjoying a life filled with hearty meals and home-baked 3-ingredient cookies. Walk into a supermarket with Inspector Gadget gear, and be ready to go through some of the ingredients and nutritional information before adding it to your cart. Whenever you reach for something you know will not contribute to your goals of enjoying a healthy life, ask yourself if those two minutes of bliss are genuinely worth the sacrifice.

Many of the previous chapters have focused on what has been holding you back, controlling and manipulating your food decisions, and keeping you stuck in an unhealthy life you have been dreading for far too long. Those are all real and important to understand. However, with the blessing of understanding comes the wisdom to choose a different path or find the right tools to fight against those forces getting in the way of your health, well-being, and fitness goals. However, you still have a significant amount of autonomy regarding what you put in your body. Despite your circumstances, childhood traumas, or the ingenuity of the men and women in white coats.

Keep a Food Diary

Journaling and keeping a food diary is an excellent first step to living healthily. "It can help you understand your eating habits and patterns and help you identify the foods — good and not-so-good — you eat regularly. Research shows that keeping a journal can be a very effective tool for people interested in losing weight to help change behavior. In one weight loss study of nearly 1,700 participants, those who kept daily food records lost twice as much weight as those who kept no records (McManus, 2019). Journaling can help you discover specific recurring patterns that contribute to unhealthy eating. If you can recognize the causes of your behavior, you are better able to manage them when they appear in the future.

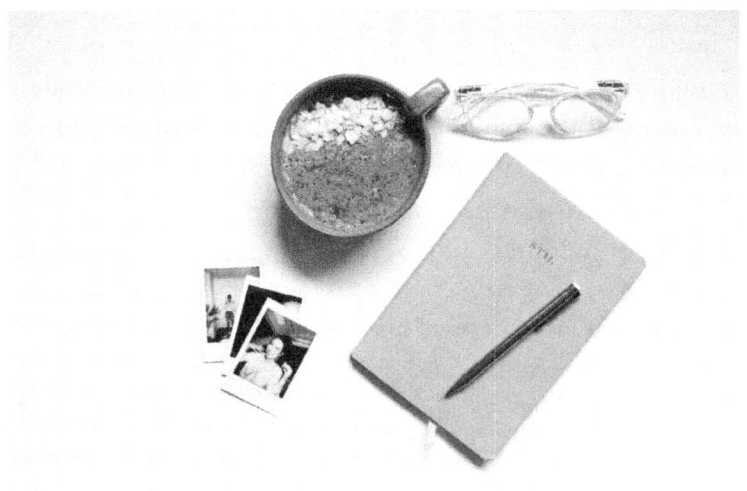

10-Day Food Journal

Over the next ten days, take note of everything you eat and drink. Even if you grab a small bite of something, jot it down. Writing the goods and volume will be beneficial when looking at your journal after ten days. However, for this to be effective, you also want to write down the following:

- **At what times did you eat?** Breakfast, lunch, and supper are likely to be there, but perhaps you may spot yourself snacking in between meals or at certain times.

- **Where did you eat?** Do you eat in the car while driving or while chilling on the couch and relaxing? Do you hover over the fridge and grab a few mouthfuls of whatever you are craving?

- **What else are you doing while eating?** Are you watching television or chatting with someone? Are you scrolling through social media?

- **Who are you eating with?** Alone or with a friend, spouse, children, or colleagues?

- **What mood are you in?** Happy, sad, bored, lonely, stressed, tired, or angry?

Carry your notebook or pad with you everywhere. You cannot trust yourself to write about it several minutes or hours later. Life can be very distracting, and you can easily forget that sip of soda you took when you stood up to stretch your legs. Try not to judge yourself during this challenge. This is not a time to take a hard look at what you are eating and feel ashamed about snacking a dozen times a day. If you judge yourself, you might not want to add all the details or could fail to complete the assessment because you are feeling guilty about it. After the ten days, see if you pick up on any patterns across the days. Do you eat more around a specific time or when you are with a particular person? Do you find yourself having more celebratory snacks or snacks to calm the nerves?

The more you understand your eating habits, the higher the chances of making changes to them. For example, suppose you know you eat a larger portion after what you have considered a stressful day when you leave the office after such a day. In that case, you can remind yourself to start the evening with a relaxing foot soak instead of having dinner as soon as you get home. If you notice you eat more when your spouse is around you, let them know that you think it would be best if the two of you tried a healthy eating challenge for several days as you need some encouragement with a new goal you have set for yourself. Some spouses or friends would be happy to join the challenge or maybe wait to eat when you are not around in an effort to support you.

Practice Mindful Eating

Mindful eating fits in with journaling and relates to what was discussed earlier on memory rehearsal. Mindful eating, however, forms part of a broader practice known as mindfulness. Mindfulness is a Zen Buddhism ritual of "paying attention in a particular way, on purpose, in the present moment, and nonjudgmentally" (Nelson, 2017). The purpose is to stay present at the moment and appreciate what the present has to offer—not concerning oneself with the future or the past. Mindfulness can be applied to any life experience, from how you eat to how you walk. With mindful eating, the goal is to enjoy whatever food you have on your plate and find a deep appreciation for it. Nevertheless, it does go beyond this and includes:

- Eating slowly and with no external distractions. No TV, no music, no podcasts. Just you and your food.

- Paying attention to hunger cues. This means eating only when you are hungry and not just in the mood for munching on something. It is also about understanding when you are full and not only looking at the plate to determine this for you.

- Involving your senses in your eating experience. Pay attention to the colors, smells, textures, sounds, and flavors.

- Eating to maintain health and well-being. Food should be seen as a way to sustain the body, not only to feed your dopamine centers.

- Understanding how food makes you feel. When you are focused, you will notice which meals make you feel happier, nostalgic, or neutral.

This is a practice that takes time to perfect and requires meticulous effort. Mindful eating is not something we are usually introduced to as children. We chat with friends and family or sit in front of the TV while eating. Even if you are alone or not distracted by anything, the goal is typically to get the food into the mouth and stomach, with little thought to the experience of the food itself. However, practicing mindful eating can bring about additional health benefits beyond the nutritional value of the healthy foods you will be eating. The more you practice this, the more mindful you will become in other areas of your life, further contributing to your overall well-being and joy.

The Raisin Test

Take one raisin (it does not matter if you enjoy these or not) and put it in front of you. Imagine you have never seen a raisin before, you have no recollection of the taste, so you do not have any judgments about whatever is in front of you. You are just looking at a small thing. Pick it up and feel its weight. Observe its surface closely—every curve, ridge, and smooth element. See if it shines if you hold it in a particular way. Smell the object—do you like how it smells? Roll it between your hands, and squeeze it gently. Does it make a sound as you press? Is it squishy, or does it remain un-squashed? How do you feel about this aspect of the object?

Place the raisin between your lips for a few seconds to see if you notice any response from your mouth, stomach, or heart. Without chewing, let the raisin roll around your mouth. How does it taste; is there a taste? Is your mouth salivating? What do you want to do with it? Take one bite, and notice how you feel. Chew some more, and pay attention to what each chew experience brings. The raisin must be totally liquefied between your tongue and teeth before swallowing it. Once you have swallowed, how do you feel about this experience with this new object?

This is what mindful eating means. It is about taking on every food experience as though it were new and paying attention to every detail about it. You do not have to touch a warm bowl of chicken stew you have made, but you will want to pay attention to every taste experience you can grab from it spoon by spoon. Preconceived ideas about what you enjoy eating and what you dislike are removed from the experience, and you are left with a plate of liquids, proteins, and vegetables, which you have to decipher with your mouth. Notice how you did not question your experiences with the raisin. There is no need to explain why you are feeling like that. You just ask how it makes you feel; answer that question, and move on.

Be Thoughtful in Choosing Your Diet

Choose a diet that works well for your body, not just one that you have heard has had an impactful result on someone else. Every person is different, and although none of us need processed foods, how we obtain our nutritional well-being will vary. It will be helpful if you keep a food diary as you do the detox so you can have reliable data available when choosing your diet. Each diet has its pros and cons, and regardless of what anyone tells you, no diet is intrinsically better than the other. Test, observe, and follow through; that is the best approach.

Thousands of diets and nutritional plans are available, each sporting its own benefits and evidence for proof of concept. However, most diets can be highly restrictive, leading to nutritional deficits, which is one of the things this book aims to avoid. The following three diets are less stringent, and people who follow these diets have seen great results in terms of their health and well-being.

- **Mediterranean Diet.** This diet is excellent for long-term health and supports heart health. Red meat, processed sugars, and processed fats are avoided. While fruits, vegetables, fish, legumes, and healthy oils (like olive oil, nuts, and avocados) are highly encouraged.

- **The Zone Diet.** It emphasizes paying close attention to what you eat and is often used to help one lose weight or maintain body fat levels. With the zone diet, you must measure the macronutrients you consume with every meal, balancing about 40% carbohydrates, 30% protein, and 30% fats. Processed foods are avoided for the most part, and emphasis is placed on healthy fats and unrefined carbs like whole grains.

- **The Pescetarian Diet**. This diet is great for inflammation, reducing joint pain experienced if you have a disease like arthritis. It has also been shown to decrease heart disease and cancer. Much like vegetarians, with the pescetarian diet, you cannot eat meat, only fish. Pay careful attention to avoiding processed foods, even if they are vegetarian or vegan-friendly.

Do Intermittent Fasting

This is not a diet, as some people consider it, but rather an eating plan or strategy. You can be vegan or follow a Mediterranean diet and still practice intermittent fasting. Some studies have found that intermittent fasting "may offer benefits such as fat loss, better health, and increased longevity. Proponents claim that an intermittent fasting program is easier to maintain than traditional, calorie-controlled diets" (Leonard, 2020). It has also been shown to reduce inflammation and reduce the risks or conditions associated with diseases that are caused by inflammation like arthritis, Alzheimer's, strokes, or multiple sclerosis.

Intermittent Fasting calls for skipping meals or eating within specific timeframes while remaining completely fasted during the other times. Those who try to argue against this strategy claim that it is terrible because it means you will not be able to have three meals and three snacks per day like we have been told to have. Yet, there is no scientific effort to support the idea that we must have multiple meals spaced throughout the day. It could even be that this was another idea brought forward to incite consumer buying behavior. Unless you have a severe medical condition, for example, but not limited to diabetes, kidney stones, or gastroesophageal reflux, for which you first need to consult your medical advisor, intermittent fasting is safe for anyone.

There are several different ways to practice intermittent fasting, depending on your current eating habits, weight loss goals, or simply what your body and mind can handle. I suggest starting with more straightforward strategies before trying to fast for more extended periods like 20-24 hours.

- **The 12:12 method.** This is the eating plan many people like to get started on when they try intermittent fasting because it is not too tricky. You are not likely to miss any meals. You will get to fast for 12 hours, then eat within the other 12 hours. So, if you have breakfast at 8 a.m., you will have your last meal before 8 p.m.

- **The 16:8 method.** Like the above, you get to fast for 16 hours, then eat within an eight-hour window. You will likely have to skip one of your meals, typically breakfast or supper. So, you can eat between 12 p.m. and 8 p.m or 8 a.m. and 4 p.m. You cannot alternate between the days; however, you must decide which meal you are willing to live without for as long as possible.

- **The 2:5 method.** This involves regularly eating for five days and fasting for two days. During fasting, you can consume a maximum amount of 500-600 calories. This can be split across two or three small foods like fruit or a salad, or you can have it as one light meal and fast for the rest of the day.

- **The 20:4 method.** This is also referred to as the warrior diet and requires you to fast for 20 hours daily. This is not a strategy that you should implement long-term. Instead, you can use it for several days at a time, reverting to other methods.

- **Alternate fasting**. Another problematic strategy to master and not suitable for long-term practice. As the name suggests, you have to alternate between the days you are fasting and the days you eat regularly. On the fasting days, you can choose to eat nothing for 24 hours or have up to 600 calories.

Something important to note here is that you would benefit greatly from consuming a lot of water during those hours when you are fasting. You can also have sugar-free tea and any other beverage that does not contain any sweeteners. Finally, during eating windows, eat reasonable portions. Do not try to make up for the calories lost, as this defeats the whole purpose of the eating strategy.

Get Rid of Sugar

No, this is not a ploy to get you to join the keto diet. By sugar, I am only referring to added sugar, particularly those found in processed foods. Fruits, some vegetables, and full-fat dairy products contain sugar. However, the volumes of sugar in these are not harmful to your body as you would find with highly palatable foods. Ice cream, milkshakes, frosted cakes, candy, and sugary soda drinks are some foods with the highest amount of refined sugar. However, there is a surprising number of foods positioned as healthy that can also contain a lot of sugar, like fruit juice, granola bars, bread, and low-fat fruit yogurt.

Getting rid of sugar will bring about specific changes to your body and mind. The experience will not be pleasurable initially, but eventually, you will adjust to the new glucose levels in your body. When you first stop eating these products, you are likely to feel exhausted, experience headaches or mental fog, and be slightly irritable. But once this wears off, you will notice:

- **Your mood will improve**. As the rush from the constant dopamine leaves your system, you are likely to feel moody and even sad. But dopamine always self-regulates and should return to baseline within a few days. Plus, the happiness and pleasure you will experience now will be more natural. You are not likely to feel fluctuating levels of joy and sadness like you would with high sugar-induced dopamine.

- **Your skin will clear up**. Processed sugars cause the body to release insulin, which causes inflammation in the cells (and the skin is made up of multiple cells). Small amounts of insulin and inflammation are not damaging. However, high volumes lead to a loss in elasticity and collagen, so you lose your natural glow and suppleness. High levels of inflammation also lead to acne and rosacea, causing pimples and redness. Say goodbye to sugar, and say goodbye to bad skin.

- **Improved sleeping patterns**. If you pair no sugar with no meals four or more hours before you sleep, you are bound to experience excellent sleep. After several weeks of living without sugar, once your body has not adjusted to the new diet and nutritional inputs, you will notice you will be able to enjoy a deeper sleep, feeling refreshed and energized to take on your day.

- **You have more potential to lose weight**. Sugar does not make you gain weight; however, sugary foods are also packed with unhealthy fats and other additives, which collectively, and in high volumes, make you gain weight. So, cutting back on cakes and burgers (that have sauces that contain sugars) will contribute to you losing weight.

Removing these foods from your diet can be difficult for some people, especially considering how addicted many people have become to them: "about 10% of the U.S. population are true sugar addicts" (Drayer, 2018, para. 2). Much like most other addictions, the best solution is to rip the band-aid off and manage the withdrawal symptoms as and when they show up. Those who are not necessarily addicted to sugar but want to limit their intake further or get rid of sugary food have discovered it does not do their gut any good. It can also take a slower approach to wean themselves off some foods and beverages permanently and only eat some other sugary products once in a while.

Imagine What You Are Consuming

When Bella started her healthy living journey, like many others, she wanted to consume less sugar. She even tried the ketogenic diet for several weeks but did not appreciate the restrictiveness of the diet. Plus, ketogenic snacks are more expensive than regular snacks, and you cannot even compensate for that with a juicy apple. After quitting that diet, she came across the 10-Day Detox plan. She made a list of foods that adversely affected her gut health (leading to bloating or cramping) and her skin (causing breakouts). One of those was soda.

Now, Bella loves soda. Her whole family did. There'd almost always be a 2 Liter in the fridge waiting to be opened. They would switch between the different flavors, which gave them a sense of refreshment, knowing their favorite beverage was there. Bella knew she would have a lot of work to do if she wanted to stop drinking soda permanently, or perhaps not as frequently. She researched sodas and discovered that besides the high sugar levels, the high acidic nature of the beverage was also causing havoc on her body from the inside. One blog she came across mentioned that drinking a glass of soda is like pouring battery acid down your throat.

That is precisely the imagery Bella needed to stop drinking soda. Every time she would pour herself a glass (after meals, as a snack, or to quench her thirst), she would actively imagine that this was not a sweet and sparkling beverage but rather a battery acid. She would imagine that behind all that sugar is a bitter concoction frying her insides. After a while, the very thought of soda could not bring feelings of pleasure to her mind or her senses. Bella discovered that she holds the power to decide what tastes good and what does not. Imagining something she enjoyed broken down into its raw components made giving up on those products much more effortlessly.

Have a Cup of Coffee

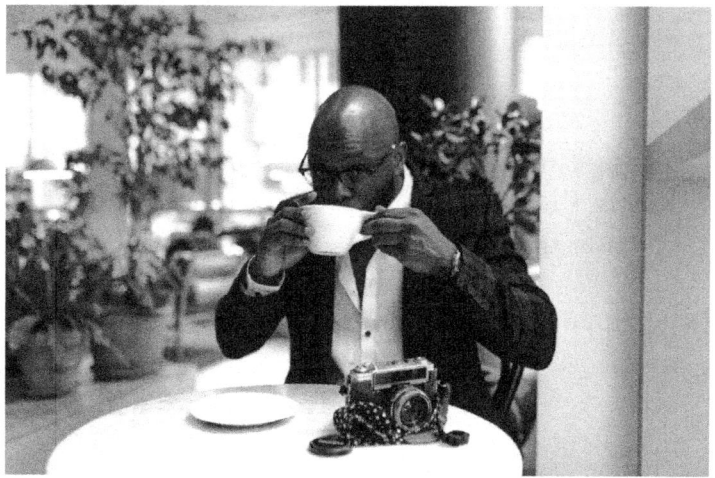

Coffee is one of those drinks that get split attention; some people love it, others not so much. If you are one of those people who cannot start your day without a cup of coffee, you may have an excellent reason to continue on that path. If you are not a coffee fan, perhaps you might want to reconsider your choice unless it is a medical concern, of course. You can also have other caffeinated drinks like tea, but that includes a considerably low volume of caffeine. The research I will be revealing below does not make many comparisons between coffee and tea, but seeing that coffee has higher volumes of caffeine and antioxidants, you would need to drink more cups of tea to receive similar benefits to the two four cups of coffee the research suggests.

One interesting reason coffee is good is that it can help you enjoy your healthy food more. Although drinking coffee does not increase your dopamine levels, coffee in itself does not make you feel happy. It does enhance how much you enjoy other things. This might be why people can wake up grumpy, have a cup, and suddenly relax into the world. According to health blogger and dietician Rachel Link (2022), other benefits of this hot beverage are:

- **It maintains brain health**. The research has mainly focused on protecting neurodegenerative diseases like Alzheimer's and Parkinson's. Across 11 studies, results showed that people who consumed more coffee had a lower chance of getting Alzheimer's. A review of 13 studies concluded that regular caffeine consumption decreased the person's risk of getting Parkinson's and slowed the progression of the disease over time.

- **It supports heart health**. Various research studies have revealed that drinking coffee can benefit the heart. One study showed that three to five cups of coffee daily reduced the risk of heart disease by 15%. Another study found that drinking three to four cups per day lowered the risk of stroke by 21%. One more study showed a significant decrease in the risk of heart failure among coffee drinkers.

- **It protects the liver**. A study revealed that drinking one cup of coffee daily lowered the risk of cirrhosis by 15%, whereas drinking four cups daily reduced the risk by 71%. In another study, it was found that in people with cirrhosis, drinking two cups of coffee per day slowed down the progression of the disease (less scarring development) as well as the progression of cancer in the liver (slower growth of mutated cells).

- **It reduces the risk of type 2 diabetes.** Research has found that with each cup of coffee a person drank, their risk of type 2 diabetes decreased by 6%. The assumption is that the high antioxidant levels in caffeine act as a countereffect on insulin.

- **It reduces the risk of depression.** A study showed that drinking four cups of coffee each day significantly reduced one's risk of becoming depressed compared to drinking only one cup. Research has also found that with each cup of coffee, the risk of being depressed was lowered by 8%. A final study to note here is that coffee consumption was also linked to a lower risk of suicide.

- **It promotes longevity.** Drinking coffee has been positively correlated with health benefits, potentially increasing one's lifespan. A review of 40 studies concluded that people who drank two to four cups of coffee per day were at a lower risk of death, regardless of age, weight, and alcohol consumption.

- **It helps with weight management.** Several studies have revealed that higher levels of coffee consumption led to lower body fat levels in men and women. Another study showed that drinking two cups of coffee per day increased the likelihood of meeting daily recommended physical activity levels by 17%.

- **It increases energy levels.** Caffeine acts as a stimulant for the central nervous system. A study that confirms this found that coffee consumption increased the time it took for participants in a cycling race to feel tired by 12%. Another study revealed that drinking coffee before and during a golf game improved the players' performance and made them feel less tired and subjectively more energized.

- **It enhances performance**. Caffeine is reported to have an ergogenic (performance-enhancing) effect. A report of 12 studies revealed that drinking coffee before exercise made participants feel more robust and helped them stick to the routine longer than the group that did not drink coffee.

Do Not Forget to Exercise

You cannot outrun a bad diet, but exercise is crucial to a healthy life. Exercise and nutrition have this interdependent relationship where one can impact and improve the other. A study by Joo et al. observed that "the 15-week exercise training appeared to motivate young adults to pursue healthier dietary preferences and to regulate their food intake" (2019, p. 1681). Most people who start exercising, especially vigorous training, do not want to counteract their workout by eating foods they know will be bad for their body. On the other hand, eating healthy does not necessarily encourage people to want to exercise (unless they are looking to lose a lot of weight fast). However, eating healthy is essential to exercise because your body will need macronutrients for energy and micronutrients to heal itself.

The type of exercise you do is important (for better healthy outputs). However, it is also vital to do physical activity that you will enjoy, so you always feel motivated to work out. When you enjoy the exercise, you are engaged. This increases your dopamine levels. So, this is another way to feel great that does not involve putting something bad into your body. That being said, here are three exercises I will recommend for anyone who does not have an activity in mind and want the best results:

- **Jogging**. This is the quickest and easiest way to get into the exercise game. You only need a basic pair of running shoes, and you are good to go. Many people worry that they will have to pay a gym membership fee and travel to and from the gym if they want to start working out. The reality is, that is an excuse, and the best gym is the ground beneath your feet. Jogging is excellent for cardiovascular activity; it helps the heart pump blood more effectively and can tone your whole body.

- **Weight exercises**. Buy several sets of dumbbells and perform weight lifting exercises in the comfort of your home. If you are comfortable heading to the gym, you can also use a wide range of weight lifting equipment. Many people always wonder if they should lift weights or do cardio like jogging, the answer is both. However, if you could only do one due to time constraints, you would benefit more from just lifting weights. Weight lifting helps you burn fat faster and build muscle in the process. If you include some bodyweight activities like split jumps and push-ups, you get some cardio benefits too.

- **Yoga**. This is an excellent activity for the body and the mind. Yoga helps you build your mindfulness and is perfect for posture, balance, and flexibility, often neglected in typical exercise routines. Plus, if you perform more high-intensity yoga workouts, you can also get some weight loss benefits. Yoga requires a lot of control and bodyweight strength, making it an excellent physical activity to begin with if you have never performed much physical activity in a long while.

More Key Tips That We Take for Granted

Although it has been highly beneficial in many respects, modern living has caused us to deviate from what the human body was designed to withstand and enjoy. This is not just about the foods we eat, but how much we move, work, and interact with others. So, if you want to be healthy, you have to take on a more holistic approach and focus on all the elements that will improve your well-being, not just nutrition and exercise—which are often the sole focus of most people. Other health tips you will benefit from include:

- **Drinking enough water.** Drinking water helps to prevent infections, deliver essential nutrients to your cells, lubricate the joints, and help all the organs, especially the brain, function better. Most people stay hydrated with sodas and fruit juices laden with sugar and, as we have established, not good for the body. After quitting these drinks, it also seems that some people would rather not drink anything instead of getting enough pure water into their system.

- **Getting enough sleep.** Quality sleep also plays a role in weight management, as well as fighting off infections and illnesses like diabetes and heart disease. Not exposing your eyes to bright light between 10 p.m. and 4 a.m. will improve the quality of your sleep, helping you think better, stress less, and improve your relationships with others.

- **Making time for family and friends.** Interpersonal relationships have been on the back burner with the rise of technology and all things digital. But connecting with humans in real time helps fight feelings of loneliness and depression. Getting social with people who love you eases anxiety and stress.

- **Staying away from drugs and alcohol**. The devastating impact of drugs and alcohol and smoking cigarettes (now vaping) will likely require a book of its own. Your health and well-being will change drastically should you stay far away from these sources of destruction. A moderate amount of wine can be heart-healthy, but if you are going to be tempted to gargle down the whole bottle, it is best just to stay away.

- **Getting a complete health checkup**. People only go to the doctor when they feel sick or have collapsed on the floor somewhere and have been driven there by someone else. When it comes to well-being, prevention is always better than cure. So, instead of waiting for something to go wrong, make an appointment with a general practitioner once a year (if you are feeling well) and get a complete body checkup. If anything seems out of balance, you can deal with it in the early stages.

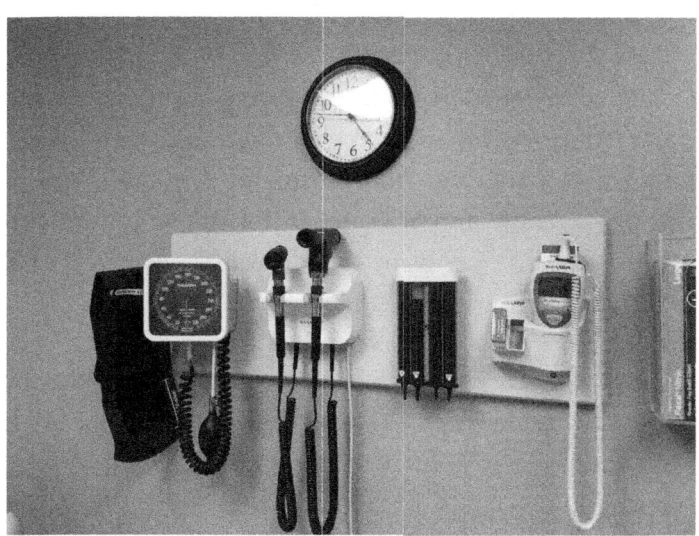

Key Takeaways

- Some practical steps you can take toward healthy living start with a food journal, documenting your current state, and moving into the lifestyle you wish to sustain. Upon completing a 10-day food diary, you will be able to tell which foods make you feel better, and you can choose a diet based on these. Mindful eating will help you appreciate healthy eating more, contributing to weight loss and health goals. Practicing intermittent fasting also has an array of benefits that you might want to consider on your journey. Finally, consider getting rid of all refined sugars; imagine what you are really eating or drinking instead of the visible, sweet-tasting treat.

- Make a cup of coffee or a four-part of your daily routine. Coffee or high amounts of caffeine can benefit your heart, brain, and liver health. It protects your body from diseases, encourages weight loss, and increases performance.

- Push yourself to exercise as part of your new healthy lifestyle. Exercise can promote healthy eating as most people feel more motivated to eat well when they are busily engaged in physical training. You must find a workout routine that you will enjoy and stick to, but some of the best physical activities you may want to get yourself involved in include jogging, weight lifting, and yoga.

- Take a holistic approach to your health. Nutrition and exercise only make up a fragment of healthy living. Hydration, sufficient sleep, no drugs and alcohol, as well as social support are just as key to enjoying your life and ensuring your longevity on this Earth.

CONCLUSION

What is the one thing you have read in this book that you believe will stick with you throughout the rest of your life? You know, that one message you will repeat to your friends when they need a little encouragement or say to yourself to keep you motivated when something on your path to healthy living is not going as intended. Each of you may have a different take-home, but when I first decided to write this book, I wanted to highlight choice. Passively living and having others determine what our lives will look like has never been a personal interest of mine. Falling victim to their circumstances and do not fully understand how they can choose not to be the victim.

Previously, I could not correctly articulate my thoughts without appearing condescending or outright rude. In this world of body positivity and embracing self-love and whatnot, we have had to be careful how we use our words even when giving advice that could potentially save the other person's life. Writing this book has made it possible to get my message across, with research and facts to back me up. It has helped me understand people better and see where their pain lies and what is holding them back from making the necessary changes. I hope you will be able to witness your experiences in this book and open your eyes to what is happening within and around you.

So, as we bring this book to a close, I want you to remember that despite your current circumstances, you hold the mental and physical capacity to bring about change to your life (and hopefully the lives of your family and friends too). The brain is able to handle much more than what you currently require of it. With the right push and food, you are bound to see changes in yourself that you would never have imagined. These changes will not come about overnight, just like your current state is an accumulation of all your thoughts, behavior, and experiences over the past years. However, once they do settle in, you will realize what you have been missing out on all these years.

I want to end this book by highlighting three essential elements to this book:

1. What has been keeping you stuck in your current unhealthy state and preventing you from eating healthy and taking care of your body?
2. The consequences of not making the necessary changes and ignoring your health can affect your life.
3. What should you do to change your lifestyle and improve your livelihood before it is too late?

What Has Been Keeping You Stuck

Unhealthy living comprises several factors that make the unhealthy state comfortable and challenging to get out of, and suddenly the healthy state does not feel urgent or even necessary. There is a lot of guilt and shame in being unable to lose weight. Or finding yourself craving and eating processed foods when you are supposed to be on a nutrition-restrictive diet. Although you should learn how to practice self-control, you do not want to be too harsh on yourself when this occurs. There is no upside to feeling ashamed of your eating habits or weight; this only brings about more unhealthy behavior and habits. For instance, you could start believing the nasty things you say to yourself, which only leads to you wanting more unhealthy foods to make yourself feel better after you have told yourself to feel shoddy. Learning to understand what is driving your unhealthy food choices is a better solution. It could be any combination of the following:

- The food industry is designed to make unhealthy foods taste extremely good. Scientists, engineers, and neurologists are hired to create and test food that will leave consumers craving more. There are approximately 16 food attributes that get considered and introduced into unhealthy foods, making them almost impossible to resist.

- The thing about delicious food is that it releases dopamine, a hormone in the brain associated with pleasure and motivation. The release and depletion of high dopamine levels make you want that activity or product more. Some people can develop food addictions that are just as strong and controlling as drug addictions.

- Another thing about these dopaminergic foods is that anything that does not make you feel good (so more bland-tasting foods, even junk food that is not as great) will now taste unnoticeable. You may develop a sort of dislike for them.

- Taste aside, unhealthy foods are more affordable than healthy foods. Preparing them is also more convenient as they come ready-made or simply need a little defrosting and heating for you to enjoy them. This is a highly convenient gesture for people who do not have time (or think they do not have time).

- When considering food and preparation, we also have to consider that we do not always eat alone or prepare food for ourselves. Food is a highly social activity, and big food companies have catered to this need. If your family, spouse, or closest friends will not be going on a diet with you, this will make it very difficult to change your current eating habits.

- One last thing to consider here is that we hold ourselves back when changing our habits. Believing things like "healthy eating is difficult" or "I am meant to be fat, it is genetic" makes you want to reinforce those ideas within your behavior. This is so you do not try hard enough to avoid processed foods.

Which one of these has been holding you back? Now that you know what is keeping you stuck, you can put in the effort to ensure you get unstuck. It is not easy fixing something when you do not know the cause, but when you have a reference, you can look for the right solutions. If you do not, you will find yourself malnourished and sickly, and death is not something that should be taken lightly.

What Could Be the Consequences

Because you would rather choose a saucy burger or thick-crusted pizza followed up with cookies and ice cream, chances are you do not get the sufficient amounts of fruits and vegetables required to sustain your body. Malnutrition is a serious condition and an after-effect of the excessive consumption of unhealthy foods. There are over 300 diseases related to this condition. If you do not make whole foods part of your dietary choices, you might soon find yourself with brittle bones, scurvy, anemia, kidney issues, or persistent skin conditions. Only fresh fruits and vegetables, whole grains, nuts and legumes, and responsibly farmed meat and meat products typically contain the right amounts of macro and micronutrients. You do not have to buy a fancy chicken wrap or be the world's best chef to consider healthy eating; you have to have a passion for life.

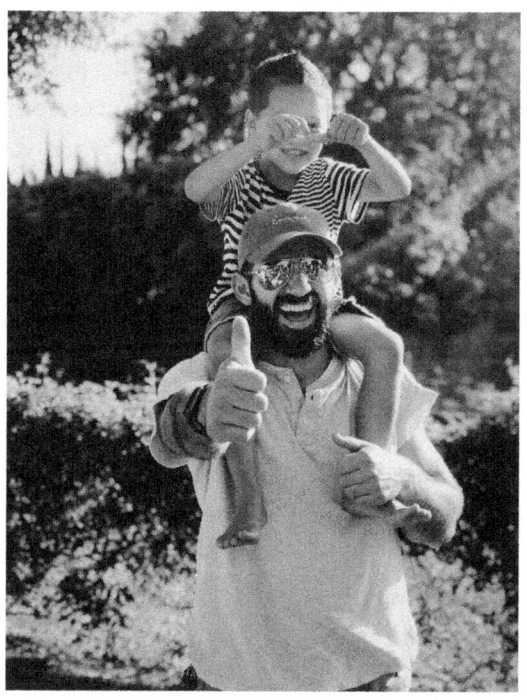

One of the biggest consequences of eating unhealthy foods is the prevalence of obesity. Sugars, salts, and fats do not necessarily make people fat. However, the overconsumption of processed foods, with excess amounts of these elements, paired with a sedentary life, eventually leads to obesity. Obesity, being overweight and undernourished, and having high volumes of waste particles (from the additives in processed foods) will put a person at risk of getting diseases such as:

- Type 2 diabetes
- Heart disease
- Alzheimer's disease
- Cirrhosis

- Cancer
- Chronic kidney disease

But it is not only about how these diseases affect your body; they also affect your livelihood and the lives of the people around you. We do not live in isolation (even if we do not necessarily have a close family). Someone will have to take care of you when you fall ill, even if they are being paid to do so.

Find a strong reason to fight for your health. It is easy to neglect your own concerns, but when you have others depending on you and your well-being, you get to think twice about ignoring your health. Your reason does not have to be a child or a spouse, it can be the fact that you would someday like to inspire millions with your story, invent something that could solve a prominent global issue, or maybe you would like to be one of the people who will colonize the planet Mars. It can be realistic or outrageous, as long as it drives you to think twice before putting another sloppy fry in your mouth.

What Power Do You Hold

It might not always feel like it, but you do hold the power to change your life, make better decisions, and engage in behavior that will boost your longevity. Enjoying food has to come from a place of enjoying life. When you appreciate all this Earth has to offer, you start to see the world and our behavior from a new perspective. There is no doubt that forces are holding you back from living a healthier life, but this can change when you:

- Become hyper-aware of your poor eating habits, and decide to make the necessary changes to start eating healthily.

- Practice mindfulness and mindful eating so you get to enjoy your healthy meals more; you remember all the positive qualities of healthy foods and feel satiated quickly, so you do not overindulge.

- Choose a nutrition plan that you will be able to commit to and which permits the consumption of all or most major food groups. Feel free to test different diets before settling on the one that works for you. Practice intermittent fasting to receive more weight loss and immune-boosting benefits.

- Reduce the amount of sugar you consume, and consider completely removing processed sugars from your diet. Sugar in processed food is highly addictive, and overconsumption of those foods leads to many health concerns you simply do not need.

- Enjoy more coffee or caffeine as part of your diet. If you are leading a reasonably healthy life, you can reduce the amount of caffeine, as you will not be concerned with the diseases coffee has been shown to fight.

- Find the time to exercise and perform physical activities that you will enjoy. Exercise has an incredible dopaminergic effect on the human mind. The feeling of pleasure from physical activity is often sustained over longer periods. For instance, it does not run out as quickly as a pack of chocolate. If you are not too picky about the type of workout, try jogging, weight lifting (with dumbbells and using your body weight), and yoga.

- Take a holistic approach to healthy living. This means you do not only focus on nutrition and exercise as most others would, but try to ensure that every aspect of your life is in check, including your sleep, emotional, and social well-being. It also means taking a preventative approach to your health by getting annual checkups.

Final Thoughts

Although I want you to remember the core teachings presented in this book, my intention is for you to come back and read some of the key takeaways or challenges. This way, you can get a refresher and remember what is required to live a healthy life and enjoy it. As humans, we often learn through repetition. So, I do not expect you to have everything on lock by next week. You will have to remind yourself every other day of the type of life you want and maybe even remind yourself why all of that is important. A friend of mine saw someone who was morbidly obese, who seemed to struggle to take each breath, and was instantly inspired to go to the gym. But the next week, that person was not there to send him a "reminder" of the body and life he did not want, so he did not go to the gym.

The teachings and warnings shared in this book are going to encourage you to take action over the next few days. However, they might not be as vivid in your memory next week. You will likely transition back to your default, with plenty of processed foods and beverages, neglecting your body and mind. We certainly do not want that. In the introduction, I encouraged you to make highlights and take notes. I hope you take that suggestion to heart, as you will be able to go back to those highlighted pages and use them as reminders of what you believe is important for you to do.

Another way you will be able to remember is if you have someone there to talk to about this book and healthy living in general. Share this book with your friends and family, so they can also access this knowledge. That way, you can ask them about some of the challenges or terms used in this book, and perhaps they will be able to give you the refresher you need. Sharing new information with others makes the lessons stick. I sincerely hope you have enjoyed reading this book and are excited to discuss it with others. If this is the case, I have a request. Kindly leave a review on Amazon. This way, others can gain this knowledge as well. Plus, if more consumers demand better food, those big food corporations will be forced to take action.

REFERENCES

Better Health Channel. (n.d.). *Cancer and food.* Better Health Channel. https://www.betterhealth.vic.gov.au/health/conditionsandtreatments/cancer-and-food#protecting-against-cancer-%E2%80%93-foods-to-%E2%80%98eat-more-of%E2%80%99

Bjarnadottir, A. (2019 May 21). *Seven nutrient deficiencies that are incredibly common.* Healthline. https://www.healthline.com/nutrition/7-common-nutrient-deficiencies

Centers for Disease Control and Prevention. (n.d.). *Only one in ten adults get enough fruits or vegetables.* Centers for Disease Control and Prevention. https://www.cdc.gov/nccdphp/dnpao/division-information/media-tools/adults-fruits-vegetables.html#:~:text=Only%201%20in%2010%20Adults,Fruits%20or%20Vegetables%20%7C%20DNPAO%20%7C%20CDC

Cleveland Clinic. (2022 March 23). *Dopamine.* Cleveland Clinic. https://my.clevelandclinic.org/health/articles/22581-dopamine

Crowe, K. (2013 March 06). *Food cravings engineered by industry.* CBC. https://www.cbc.ca/news/health/food-cravings-engineered-by-industry-1.1395225

Drayer, L. (2018 March 22). *One-month sugar detox: A nutritionist explains how and why.* CNN Health. https://edition.cnn.com/2017/06/09/health/sugar-detox-food-drayer/index.html

Gloria. (2013 October 23). *The psychology of food labeling: Read before you feed.* Life At U Of T. https://blogs.studentlife.utoronto.ca/lifeatuoft/2013/10/23/the-psychology-of-food-labeling-read-before-you-feed/

Havard School of Public Health. (2014). *Friends, family can influence your weight: For good or bad.* Harvard School of Public Health. https://www.hsph.harvard.edu/news/hsph-in-the-news/friends-and-family-can-influence-your-weight/

Higgs, S., Robinson, E. & Lee, M. (2012). *Learning and memory processes and their role in eating: Implications for limiting food intake in overeaters.* Current Obesity Reports, 1, pp. 91-98. https://doi.org/10.1007/s13679-012-0008-9

Huber, J. (2019 October 10). *Names matter: Transforming how we label foods.* Stanford Medicine. https://scopeblog.stanford.edu/2019/10/10/names-matter-transforming-how-we-label-foods/

Huberman, A. (2021). *Controlling your dopamine for motivation, focus and satisfaction.* [Video]. Andrew Huberman. [YouTube]. https://www.youtube.com/watch?v=QmOF0crdyRU&t=37s

Joo, J., Williamson, S. A., Vazquez, A. I., Fernandez, J. R. & Bray, M. S. (2019). *The influence of 15-week exercise training on dietary patterns among young adults.* International Journal of Obesity, 43, pp. 1681-1690. https://doi.org/10.1038/s41366-018-0299-3

Leonard, J. (2020 April 16). *Seven ways to do intermittent fasting.* Medical News Today. https://www.medicalnewstoday.com/articles/322293

Link, R. (2022 January 11). *Nine unique benefits of coffee.* Healthline. https://www.healthline.com/nutrition/top-evidence-based-health-benefits-of-coffee

Madhurakavi, M. (2021 April 20). *Understanding the cost of packaging.* Packmojo. https://packmojo.com/blog/understanding-packaging-pricing-economies-of-scale/

Margo, C. E. & Harman, L. E. (2016). *Autoimmune disease: Conceptual history and contributions to ocular immunology.* Survey of Ophthalmology, 61(5), pp. 680-688. https://doi.org/10.1016/j.survophthal.2016.04.006

Mayo Clinic. (2021 April 27). *Cancer.* Mayo Clinic. https://www.mayoclinic.org/diseases-conditions/cancer/symptoms-causes/syc-20370588

McCarthy, M. (2010 June 22). *Journal writing your way to healthy eating.* Create Write Now. https://www.createwritenow.com/journal-writing-blog/bid/13224/Journal-Writing-Your-Way-to-Healthy-Eating

McManus, K. D. (2019 January 31). *Why keep a food diary?* Harvard Health Publishing. https://www.health.harvard.edu/blog/why-keep-a-food-diary-2019013115855#:~:text=It%20can%20help%20you%20understand,tool%20to%20help%20change%20behavior.

Moynihan, R., Heath, I. & Henry, D. (2002). *Selling sickness: The pharmaceutical industry and disease mongering.* BMJ, 324(7342), pp. 886-891. https://doi.org/10.1136/bmj.324.7342.886

Nelson, J. B. (2017). *Mindful eating: The art of presence while you eat.* Diabetes Spectrum, 30(3), pp. 171-174. https://doi.org/10.2337/ds17-0015

Raghunathan, R., Naylor, R. W., & Hoyer, W. D. (2006). *The unhealthy = tasty intuition and its effects on taste inferences, enjoyment, and choice of food products.* Journal of Marketing, 70(4), pp. 170-184. https://www.jstor.org/stable/30162121

Raman, R. (2019 January 21). *16 healthy foods packed with umami flavor.* Healthline. https://www.healthline.com/nutrition/umami-foods

Rang, H. (2012). *Bad pharma: How drug companies mislead doctors and harm patients.* British Journal of Clinical Pharmacology, 75(5), pp. 1377-1379. https://doi.org/10.1111/bcp.12047

Robinson, E., Blissett, J. & Higgs, S. (2012). *Changing memory of food enjoyment to increase food liking, choice and intake.* The British Journal of Nutrition, 108(8), pp. 1505-1510. https://doi.org/10.1017/S0007114511007021

See, C. (2020 March 25). *The cost healthy eating versus unhealthy eating.* Plutus Foundation. https://plutusfoundation.org/2020/healthy-eating-budget/

Singh, S. P., Wal, P., Wal, A., Srivastava, V., Tiwari, R. & Sharma, R. D. (2016). *Understanding autoimmune disease: An update review.* International Journal of Pharmaceutical Technology and Biotechnology, 3(3), pp. 51-65. https://www.researchgate.net/publication/318393865_UNDERSTANDING_AUTOIMMUNE_DISEASE_AN_UPDATE_REVIEW

Spritzler, F. (2021 May 19). *21 reasons to eat real food.* Healthline. https://www.healthline.com/nutrition/21-reasons-to-eat-real-food

U.S. Right to Know. (n.d.). *Food-related diseases.* U.S. Right to Know. https://usrtk.org/food-related-diseases/

Werle, C., Trendel, O. & Ardito, G. (2013). *Unhealthy food is not tastier for everybody. The healthy = tasty French intuition.* Food Quality and Preference, 28(1), pp. 116-121. https://doi.org/10.1016/j.foodqual.2012.07.007

Witherly, S. A. (2013 November 30). *Why humans like junk food.* University Inc. Publishing. https://jamesclear.com/wp-content/uploads/2013/11/why-humans-like-junk-food-steven-witherly.pdf

WIC Nutrition Risk. (2018 June). *341 nutrient deficiency or disease.* WIC Nutrition Risk. https://health.mo.gov/living/families/wic/localagency/wom/pdf/341-definition.pdf

World Health Organization. (2021 June 09). *Obesity.* World Health Organization. https://www.who.int/news-room/facts-in-pictures/detail/6-facts-on-obesity#:~:text=At%20least%202.8%20million%20people%20each%20year%20die%20as%20a,tripled%20between%201975%20and%202016.

Images

Ayrton, A. (2021). *A blurred out woman holding an apple and a donut.* [Image]. Pexels. https://www.pexels.com/photo/woman-showing-apple-and-bitten-doughnut-6551415/

Criativithy. (2019). *Female on the road eating fruit loops.* [Image]. Pexels. https://www.pexels.com/photo/woman-sitting-on-the-road-eating-froot-loops-1805405/

Grabowska, K. (2020). *A man with a protruding belly eating a burger.* [Image]. Pexels. https://www.pexels.com/photo/man-with-hamburger-getting-his-waist-measured-5714314/

Inouye, M. (2019). *A table with a diary and pen, with glasses, coffee and photographs on the side.* [Image]. Pexels. https://www.pexels.com/photo/brown-ceramic-cup-beside-notebook-and-pen-2180092/

Kutsaiev, R. (2020). *Slices of dried citrus fruits.* [Image]. Pexels. https://www.pexels.com/photo/sliced-oranges-grapefruit-and-kiwi-fruit-3471790/

McGuire, R. (2014). *Man eating cookies looking guilty.* [Image]. Pixabay. https://pixabay.com/photos/hunger-hungry-eating-cookie-413685/

Myriams Fotos. (2016). *An image of milk and cheese.* [Image]. Pixabay. https://pixabay.com/photos/milk-cheese-cheese-slices-1385548/

Nappy. (2018). *A man sipping from a cup.* [Images]. Pexels. https://www.pexels.com/photo/man-sitting-in-front-of-round-table-while-sipping-from-white-ceramic-mug-936019/

Nelson, H. (2018). *A father and son smiling at the camera.* Pexels. https://www.pexels.com/photo/man-talking-picture-while-smiling-1456951/

PD Pics. (2013). *Frozen peas.* [Image]. Pixabay. https://pixabay.com/photos/peas-frozen-vegetables-green-raw-166969/

Piacquadio, A. (2020). *A man in bed looking sick.* [Image]. Pexels. https://www.pexels.com/photo/young-man-in-sleepwear-suffering-from-headache-in-morning-3771115/

Piacquadio, A. (2020). *Two women getting ready to eat a watermelon.* [Image]. Pexels. https://www.pexels.com/photo/photo-of-women-eating-watermelon-3760053/

Samuel, T. (2021). *Woman eating a variety of junk food.* [Image]. Pexels. https://www.pexels.com/photo/hungry-woman-eating-junk-food-6697285/

Shultz, S. (2021). *Two plus-size women in pink dresses.* [Image]. Pexels. https://www.pexels.com/photo/beautiful-plus-size-women-in-the-park-8145947/

Tankilevitch, P. (2020). *Female biting on a gummy candy.* [Image] Pexels. https://www.pexels.com/photo/woman-in-white-shirt-eating-a-gummy-candy-5469290/

Tarazevich, A. (2021). *Jars of organic turmeric and cinnamon sticks.* [Images]. Pexels. https://www.pexels.com/photo/glass-jars-with-turmeric-and-cinnamon-sticks-7771976/

TerriC. (2017). *A breakfast quiche with eggs and peppers on the side.* [Image]. Pixabay. https://pixabay.com/photos/quiche-eggs-brunch-breakfast-2067686/

Tukhfatullina, A. (2022). *A bowl of oats and berries with chia seeds.* [Image]. Pexels. https://www.pexels.com/photo/porridge-with-fresh-raspberries-11532336/

Wright, R. (2017). *Medical checkup equipment in a doctor's office.* [Image]. Pixabay. https://pixabay.com/photos/doctors-office-checkup-medical-2610509/

Wurzinger, B. (2016). *A platter of healthy foods.* [Image]. Pixabay. https://pixabay.com/photos/breakfast-healthy-hummus-spread-1804457/

We'd Like to Hear From You

The publisher invites you to share your feedback by leaving a review on our page.

We value your thoughts and testimonies as we continue to write high-quality books that help improve the lives of our readers.

If you like this book, check out our other books available on Amazon.

Printed in Great Britain
by Amazon